FINALLY

STOP

PROCRASTINATING

FINALLY

STOP

PROCRASTINATING

**When Nothing Else Works,
Unlock Your Hidden Power to Succeed**

Linda Gannaway, Ed.D.

The author gratefully acknowledges those who granted permission to use copyrighted and previously published material. A list of permissions is included at the end of this book. See the Notes section for additional information.

Also written by Linda Gannaway
The Power of Life Lessons

The purpose of this book is to help you stop procrastinating and unlock your hidden power to succeed. It is based on the author's education, experiences, and insights, along with the information she has learned from others, including her students and clients, as well as other authors, coaches, and mentors.

The author's personal stories in this book are true. The stories about other people are used to describe situations the author has encountered; however, circumstances have been changed to protect anonymity and in some cases, composites are used. Any resemblance to actual identities is unintentional.

You should use the book as a general guide and resource, but as with all books of this kind, it cannot address the individual situations of readers. It is not intended to be, nor should it be, relied on or construed as medical, health, nutritional, psychological, financial, legal, or any other kind of professional advice, service, or therapy. As noted several times in the book, you should consult a competent professional in the appropriate area for any individual advice or treatment you need.

The results you get from reading and doing the activities in the book may be different from the results others achieve. All information and references in the book are believed to be accurate at the time of publishing but may change over time. There may also be typographical and other errors in the text.

The author and publisher are not liable or responsible for any loss or damage caused, or alleged to have been caused, directly or indirectly, by the information and activities contained or referenced in this book, or your application of them.

Print ISBN: 978-0-9985066-2-3
Ebook ISBN: 978-0-9985066-7-8

First edition

Cover design: 100 Covers
Interior design and image customization: mgfdesigner.com

Dedicated to those of you who want to break free from the procrastination that has kept you from achieving your goals and dreams, that has prevented you from becoming your best self, and that has stopped you from sharing your gifts and talents and stepping into your light.

May you finally find success.

The really happy people are those who have broken the chains of procrastination, those who find satisfaction in doing the job at hand. They're full of eagerness, zest, productivity.

You can be, too.

– Norman Vincent Peale

CONTENTS

Chapter 1

Looking for Answers

The first time I remember procrastinating was when I was in the third grade. Our family used to go over to my grandparents' house—a lot. There weren't any kids my age that I could play with, so it was boring, and I usually didn't want to go.

One time I kept dragging my feet when we were getting ready to leave our house, and I made our whole family late. Everyone got mad at me, my two older sisters and my parents. Did it bother me that they were mad? Not really. In fact, it felt kind of good. I didn't realize it at the time, but it made me feel powerful to make them wait.

When I was in college, I used to put off any studying until the night before a test. Then I would stay up half the night, cram like crazy, and go take the exam. I still got good grades, so I didn't see a downside. When I was in graduate school, procrastination became a game. I would wait until the last minute to get ready to go to a class or a meeting, fly into a frenzy, sprint out the door, and make it there with maybe, *maybe* three minutes to spare. Or I would intentionally stall before paying my bills, then marvel at how I always made it on time.

So basically, I would write, direct, and star in my own self-created dramas. I felt like Wonder Woman! It was lots and lots of unnecessary stress, but it was also fun and an energy rush. That's when I started getting hooked on my own adrenaline.

Fast forward to when I got my first full-time job as a counselor at a university counseling center. After years of graduate coursework and internships, I finally landed my dream job, and I loved it. Only I started actually being late to staff meetings. No one said anything to me, but they noticed. Here I was, early on in my career, and I was jeopardizing my professional reputation. I knew it was unprofessional, disrespectful, and downright rude. It definitely wasn't fun, and it wasn't a game anymore. But I couldn't stop. And I didn't understand why.

Then one day, I went to a staff meeting—predictably late—and the only empty chair was clear across the room. I panicked and tried to slink to my seat like I was invisible, but I could feel everyone's eyes watching me as I made that long walk across the floor. I didn't even look up when I got to my seat. I felt so humiliated. It was horrible.

After that meeting, I went back to my office, closed the door, sat down in my chair, and for the first time ever, seriously asked myself, "Why am I always late?" And from deep inside came this answer, "Because it feels powerful."

So that was it. This was just like me in the third grade, feeling powerful when I made other people wait on me. I felt incredibly immature and embarrassed. But it also made perfect sense. I had been a psychology major in college, and in my very first class we learned that if you keep doing something over and over, it's because there is a reward or a payoff. You're getting something out of it. If there is no reward, you'll stop doing it. If it's not meeting a need or a desire, you won't continue.

Then I thought *Wait a minute. We all want to feel powerful. There's nothing wrong with that.* But I needed to learn healthy ways to feel powerful. So I started getting really good at my job and finding more ways to feel competent in my personal life. Then I didn't have such a strong reason to procrastinate, and it started to lose its grip on me.

My epiphany after that staff meeting was a turning point, and my life gradually got better and better. I still procrastinated on certain things, and sometimes I barely met my deadlines. But my eyes were wide open. I knew exactly what I was doing, and I didn't get stuck in my delays the way I had before. After a long and productive career, I retired from my last university position and wrote my first book, *The Power of Life Lessons*, which includes lessons on procrastination. I spoke on procrastination and did life coaching with people who were struggling the same way I had. I felt like I was living my dream life, until . . .

The bottom fell out. I suddenly lost my momentum, ran into mental roadblocks, and found myself procrastinating in several areas of my life. My stuckness felt deep and unyielding, and it acted like a noose around my neck that would tighten every time I started moving toward my goals. Here I was once again. After more than twenty-five years of working as a counselor, hypnotherapist, and university instructor, I felt like I should be way past this nonsense. Yet I was still struggling. I became obsessed with figuring out why.

Part of my motivation was wanting to achieve some goals I'd had in the back of my mind for a long time, goals that were bigger, riskier, and scarier than anything I had ever done before. Those goals began to feel heavy, and I either needed to accomplish them or make a decision to mark them off my mental to-do list. I knew I would regret it if I didn't at least try to reach my goals, so I kept searching for answers.

Another aspect of my motivation was wanting to be able to respect myself and feel proud of who I was as a person. Procrastination was stealing part of my self-esteem. I got tired of being disappointed with myself, and I didn't want to look back when I was eighty-five years old and feel apologetic about my life.

Finally Breaking Free

I had already found most of the skills needed to stop procrastinating, and those worked well for many years. But during the same time as when I fell back into my procrastination, I got certified as a life coach. While doing that training, I realized I still had **internal blocks** that had been silently holding me back my whole life. These blocks mainly consisted of limiting beliefs, things I had unconsciously been telling myself again and again. Things like *Don't be too powerful* and *Don't outshine others*. Broad, oppressive beliefs that put the brakes on all kinds of forward movement. I already knew I had some of those beliefs. But thankfully, I learned a life coaching technique that helped me change those beliefs to empowering ones. It's the same technique that has helped thousands of people around the world do the same, with all kinds of limiting beliefs. It gets to the root cause of people's internal blocks and it releases them, sometimes in a surprisingly short period of time.

I started using that coaching technique with myself and others. I combined it with new information from brain research, along with principles from psychology on how to change habits. Putting all of that together meant I finally had all the puzzle pieces needed to keep procrastination from sabotaging my success. That's when I decided to write this book. The tools and strategies I describe have accelerated how fast I reach my goals, made me much happier, opened my life to endless possibilities, and ignited a burning passion inside of me to do more and more. This has been the case for me, as well as for my clients and many others who have also learned these strategies.

Now I'm on a mission to offer those same results and opportunities to as many people as I can. Once you learn the strategies, you can take action on your goals and dreams and start to make them happen. In the bigger scheme of things, you can finally do what you came here to do and live the life you were meant to live. Without regrets. And here's why.

After teaching classes on procrastination to literally thousands of university students, I discovered two types of procrastinators: those who are **situational procrastinators** and those who are considered **chronic procrastinators**. People who are situational procrastinators get stuck in only a few areas of their lives, often because they don't have the knowledge or skills to complete the tasks. For instance, some of my students could learn time management skills, practice a little, and then they were fine. They made their to-do lists, scheduled activities in their calendars, and took action on their goals without a lot of internal resistance. In contrast, chronic procrastinators put off doing things in many different areas of their lives and stay stuck for years, even if they know how to get them done. I could teach the students who were chronic procrastinators all kinds of techniques to manage their time but that didn't help, and they would continue to put things off.

If your procrastination has become not just a habit, but a lifestyle, or if your delays have resulted in negative consequences too many times, it's probably because—like me and other chronic procrastinators—you have internal blocks. You can't just *do* things differently like the experts advise. In spite of your best intentions, and regardless of your best efforts, you can't simply change your behavior and become more productive, because inner blocks are stopping you. And unfortunately, these blocks are usually invisible. You can't see them, touch them, feel them. You don't even consciously know what they are, which makes it all that much more difficult to change. Your blocks have a hold on you, and they won't let go.

Right now, you may feel confused by your procrastination. Overwhelmed. Helpless. Guilty. These feelings are common. After trying to fight an invisible enemy for years, some procrastinators give up hope and resign themselves to a life that is mediocre in comparison to the life of their dreams. I understand. I almost gave up. More than once.

It is important to know that your procrastination doesn't mean you are lazy or unmotivated, or that you're "one of those people" who just can't develop self-discipline. If you are still stuck, please understand there is nothing wrong with you. It's not your fault. The fault lies with your approach, with the *way* or *ways* you may have tried to stop procrastinating before now. The strategies you've been using haven't worked. **You need new strategies in order to get the results you want.**

Brain research tells us that because of competing parts of the brain, we're hardwired to procrastinate. But with the more recent scientific understanding about how the brain works, you can figure out what is holding you back. For chronic procrastinators, that sometimes means releasing parts of your inner blocks. Sometimes it means using brain hacks to "slip through the back door," to bypass your resistance in order to move forward. You may need to try several different approaches, but now it's entirely possible to find techniques that work for you.

One of my favorite sayings by best-selling author Louise Hay is,

I choose to make my future the best part of my life.

What if you could stop procrastinating and actually make that quote come true for you? What if the best of your life lies just ahead in your not-too-distant future? The following pages show you step by step how to replace your stubborn habits of waiting and backtracking with new habits that help you get more done in less time. When that happens, you'll discover a new-found confidence that helps you achieve the levels of success and happiness you want and deserve. That little voice inside of you is right when it says, "I can do better than this. I know I can. There's gotta be a way."

Will reading this book ensure that you'll never procrastinate again? Probably not. But even if you occasionally put something off, you can stop feeling bad about yourself. And if you get stuck, you will know ways to get unstuck. You can definitely learn how to procrastinate less and less, become more productive in general, and achieve more of your goals. Plus, you can start to take advantage of opportunities that may be passing you by right now because of your delays.

The hope you feel is what made you start reading this book. You *can* overcome your procrastination and start to move forward in your life, feeling excited by the progress you're making.

You have a lot to look forward to. Let's get started.

Chapter 2

The Good News About Procrastination

I'll never forget the time I just sat in my junior high school math class when we were supposed to be working on an assignment. My teacher walked by and noticed I was basically doing nothing, and she told me I had to go to early morning study hours to make up for the time I'd wasted. And she said it in front of the whole class. Talk about embarrassing. Or the time later in my life when I planned to visit a friend who lived out of town. From out of nowhere, I suddenly decided it was a good idea to vacuum my house right before I left. Somewhere in the back of my mind I knew that cleaning my house would make me late, which it did. But for some reason, I couldn't finish packing my car and get on the road.

In looking back on experiences like that, when it came to doing certain things, it felt like I would run into this massive, rock-solid wall. But that wall was inside of me. I couldn't *do* things like the math assignment, no matter how hard I tried. Even though I *wanted* to do those things and I knew *how*, I couldn't MAKE myself do them.

I talk with a lot of procrastinators and many of them tell me some version of, "I feel like I'm going through life with one foot on the gas pedal and one foot on the brakes." They say a part of them wants to get things done, but another part seems bound and determined to stop that from happening. They understand *they* are the ones putting on the brakes. And yes, they are understandably frustrated.

What about you? What's hard for you to get done? It's common for people to procrastinate on things like organizing their finances, losing weight, or even taking vacations. Or maybe you're like most other people who set New Year's resolutions, but you give up on them after two or three weeks. Like many others, you may also try to console yourself by saying something like, "Oh, well. I can always do those things later."

Or maybe instead, you are what's called a **successful procrastinator.** You wait until the last minute to get things done but still manage to meet your deadlines. For example, you fill your time doing other things instead of working on a big project. The time you have left to get it done is running out. Several nights in a row, you wake up with a jolt of anxiety in the pit of your stomach and wonder if this time, you've cut it too close. Finally, you get started and work on the project almost nonstop. You may have to stay up late, scramble to get it finished, and even then, barely turn it in on time. But what a relief when it's done. It may not be your best work, but hey, you met your deadline. You may tell yourself that the extra stress in your life was just a small price to pay for your unnecessary delays. At the same time, you may vow that you will never procrastinate again. This may seem like an extreme example, but it's the way many procrastinators live their lives.

Some procrastinators don't feel that bad when their own plans get derailed or when they derail someone else's. Or at least that's how they act. You could be the kind of procrastinator, however, who takes things to heart and regrets not following through on your promises. The time you were embarrassingly late to your cousin's wedding still makes you feel awful, especially since now she will barely speak to you. If you're like most procrastinators, you may also feel genuinely mystified about why you can't change your self-defeating behavior.

Before you become too discouraged and accept the fact that you will always procrastinate, keep reading.

The really good news is that procrastination is learned.

No one is born a procrastinator. You didn't come into this life with some genetic code that makes you put things off. Somewhere along the way, you learned to procrastinate, and you can learn to replace it with productive habits instead. The new frontier in brain research focuses on **neuroplasticity**, which describes how adaptable our brains are at changing and becoming healthier and more efficient, no matter how old we are. We just need to give our brains the right support and experiences in order to change and heal. We now know that our brains can heal from physical injuries, emotional trauma, years of bad habits, severe memory problems—even Alzheimer's. There's lots of hope for procrastinators as well.

Every time you make a promise to yourself or others and don't deliver, it takes a toll on your self-confidence. The sooner you learn how to replace your procrastination with productive habits, the quicker you get to start feeling better and finding the success that's been so elusive before now. And because of certain chemicals in your brain, even a little progress on your goals can make you feel happy and more motivated to keep going.

Today I call myself a "recovering procrastinator." After years of last-minute dashes to the finish line, I realized I no longer wanted the extra stress and back-and-forth internal conflict that my dawdling created. Nothing about it felt fun anymore. The adrenaline rush needed to pull off miraculous feats in the final hours left me feeling tired and depleted. Something inside of me shifted, and I much preferred to feel grounded, steady, and in control, easily meeting my deadlines not just on time, but ahead of time.

Plus, all of that inner conflict and the extra energy it required was getting in the way of some of my more important big goals. I knew there was more to life than what I was living, and I wanted to enjoy it while I could. Deep down inside, I also knew that if I really put my mind to it, I could get past my procrastination and start to enjoy more of my naturally powerful potential. That I could get stronger and become more of the best version of myself. So after years of struggling, I'm beyond grateful that I found what works for me. That now I rarely procrastinate and when I do, I have lots of techniques and strategies that keep me from staying stuck.

The key to my second and final procrastination turnaround was figuring out how to release my inner blocks. Now I want to help other procrastinators do the same, without having to go through the time it took and the trial-and-error experiences I went through. Because I learned how to take my foot off the brakes, I know firsthand how much better life can be. Now, instead of wondering if I will ever achieve my goals, I ask myself, "How fast can I let myself go?" and "How good can I let my life get?" I want that for you as well. In the following pages, I give you the answers that took me so long to find.

It's time for you to start listening to that little voice inside that keeps saying, "Why can't I be like people who are successful? When is it going to be my turn?" It *is* your turn. This is your chance to finally win the inner battle that has kept you from succeeding before now. Keep reading to find out what you've been up against and why your procrastination hasn't been your fault. Part of your success will come from understanding what is going on in your mind and why that has kept you stuck for so long.

What is the Inner Game of Procrastination?

Throughout this book, I will refer to the **Inner Game** of procrastination. I will explain the Inner Game in more detail in the next chapter but briefly, it's what goes on inside your brain when you procrastinate. Sometimes this mental activity is called **mindset**, or your beliefs, thoughts, emotions, and attitudes. I will use all of these terms interchangeably throughout this book, but I will call it the Inner Game more often, because that highlights the competition between different parts of your brain when you try to do certain tasks.

Just like in sporting events, this Inner Game usually has a winner and a loser at the end of the competition, only it is played completely in your head. The players in the game are first of all, your conscious mind—what you are aware of. The other players in this competition are all the other parts of your brain that can sabotage what your conscious mind wants to do. These players include the internal blocks that most people aren't aware of even when they get in the way of accomplishing a goal. These blocks live in your subconscious mind, hidden from your conscious awareness. But they become your primary "opponents" in the Inner Game. The conscious part of you wants to "win" the game by getting something done, but your subconscious mind seems to be saying, "No way!"

The subconscious part can make you come up with all kinds of distractions and excuses that keep you from focusing on your goal. You may end up feeling bamboozled when this happens, like you just got taken for a ride. You can't believe you just wasted all that time on social media—again—especially when your big project is due in two days.

So what are these internal blocks? They mainly consist of fears and limiting beliefs that we learned before the age of six from the people around us, usually our parents and other family members. The beliefs we learn from our childhood experiences are simply thoughts about reality that have become cemented into hard-and-fast truths in our minds, and we tend to accept them without question. For example, some parents tell their children they are worthy and capable. But sometimes children get messages, in various ways, that they are unworthy and incompetent. These messages can turn into beliefs about ourselves and get stored in our subconscious mind. They often continue to control us throughout our lives because they are usually silent and invisible. It's like you downloaded a software program onto your computer, and then you forgot you saved it on your hard drive.

Our limiting beliefs can create conflicts around the goals we set later in life, which then cause an internal battle, a mental tug-of-war. Maybe you want to do something that would show you are worthy and capable. If that contradicts what you learned as a child, your subconscious programming can kick in and either slow you down or stop you from taking action. You may feel resistant when you start to work on your goal and can't understand why you are suddenly anxious, tired, or just "not in the mood." It is probably because you're about to do something that goes against a belief that is a part of your invisible blocks.

Many experts agree that **at least 80 percent of the obstacles we face in life have to do with mindset, with the Inner Game,** with our subconscious, internal conflicts. On some level, you may already realize that you are your biggest obstacle to success. That you are the one getting in your own way. That you keep sabotaging the very goals you say you want to achieve. Wouldn't it feel liberating if you could learn how to win the Inner Game and stop fighting against yourself? Then you would never have a reason to say, "I'm my own worst enemy."

There's an Inner Game of Procrastination, and There's an Outer Game

Sometimes procrastinators will think: *If I just had more time, I could get more done.* Or *If I just had more money, I could accomplish my goals.* Time and money are part of the **Outer Game** of procrastination, where you "win" over all the external opponents in your environment. Outer Game opponents are anything outside of yourself that could become an obstacle in reaching a goal. Your success depends on whether you can prevent these external factors from getting in the way. Besides time and money, these opponents can include having a place to work on your goals, finding childcare, or getting up to speed with skills like time management and goal setting. The list of potential Outer Game obstacles depends on your individual circumstances at the time you want to achieve a particular goal. But basically, they consist of time, money, a suitable workspace, knowledge, skills, possibly technology support, staff or other people, and any other external resources you might need.

Most of us can find ways to work around the external obstacles we face, even when they feel impossible in the moment. We may have to wait for the right timing, but usually we can get creative, do some problem solving, and come up with a plan. If you think back on what seemed like a solid external roadblock to a goal you wanted to achieve, you may remember that you eventually found a way around it. But these Outer Game obstacles are normally less than 20 percent of what's holding us back. Usually it's the other 80-plus percent—the Inner Game blocks—that make us continue to procrastinate. We can't do problem-solving with our internal opponents if we don't even know what they are. So we keep overeating, spending too much time on our phones, or keep running late.

Most books and online advice about procrastination focus on the Outer Game. They provide external strategies aimed at changing your behavior and *doing* things differently: identify your priorities, complete your priorities through small action steps, then reward yourself. Much of the published information is excellent, and judging from the online reviews, this material helps many people beat their habit and turn into non-procrastinators who are happier and more productive.

Through teaching university classes on procrastination and time management for decades, I learned that this published material is a great fit for most situational procrastinators who are temporarily stuck. They just need to learn time management and self-management skills, and they're good to go. They use those skills to complete their goals in a reasonable amount of time, without a struggle. They follow the advice for how to play the Outer Game, change their behavior, and "win" by achieving what they want. These procrastinators usually need to go through a learning curve to become successful, so it doesn't happen overnight. And they may not be 100 percent successful all the time. But in general, they're able to take action on their goals and keep moving forward in their lives.

For a certain group of long-term, chronic procrastinators, however, suggesting external strategies and asking them to change their behavior doesn't work. Some people who procrastinate can't "win" by using Outer Game techniques. Their invisible, subconscious blocks keep their self-defeating behaviors alive and well, regardless of negative consequences and even when they have Outer Game techniques that could help. I know. I was one of them.

We live our lives in the now of present moments. If your present moments are even partially filled with avoidance, delays, stalling, and back-tracking, then you will limit your ability to accomplish your goals and enjoy your life. However, once you learn how to win the Inner Game of procrastination, what's so remarkable is that you can apply the same techniques to any and every other part of your life where you have internal blocks. It can improve the overall quality of your life in fascinating and completely unexpected ways. Ways that can lead to more opportunities. Better choices. Greater freedom. A new and improved life. And a happier you.

Guilt Doesn't Help

One time I was presenting a workshop on procrastination at a conference for college students. Just before we got started, a young woman walked in, sat down in the first row of seats, looked straight at me, and said, "You're not going to make us feel guilty, are you?" The young woman was expressing what most procrastinators think and feel. They know they struggle to get things done on time (or at all), and it makes them feel guilty. Inside, they may call themselves lazy, unmotivated, undisciplined. Chronic procrastinators, in particular, are often extremely hard on themselves.

But procrastination isn't a character problem. Your procrastination is usually caused by invisible, competing parts of your brain. And besides that, mentally beating yourself up makes it harder to change. Guilt, shame, and name-calling make you feel worse and tend to keep you stuck. You can use the energy you spend berating yourself to move forward, so no guilt trips, please.

Guilt doesn't help, but self-compassion does. As an example, when college students were told to forgive themselves for their low grades on a test, they did better on the next test than the students who were told nothing. For right now, try forgiving yourself for all the times you fell into the procrastination trap. As you will see in this book, you probably didn't know how to do things any differently. You repeated the same habits that had been going on with you for a long time, maybe years, and had no way to prevent that from happening.

Regardless of what it might look like to others, you may really try to do better. You probably want to be on time and may give that a lot of effort. You buy the latest organizer. You work on self-discipline. You swear you will never be late again. But despite your best intentions, your self-defeating patterns continue. Most procrastinators long to feel "normal," to just get things done like other people do, without turning them into some big ordeal. But when that doesn't happen, besides berating themselves, they often start to feel weak and inadequate, like they have some fatal flaw.

Worse yet, they take on "I'm a procrastinator" as part of their identity, as if it's gospel truth. Your identity, or who you believe you are as a person, directs and determines the majority of your behavior. That means you need to be very careful about how you label or describe yourself, because it will tend to become a self-fulfilling prophecy. **Procrastination is a behavior. It is something you do. It is not who you are.** When I refer to people as procrastinators in this book, it is meant to describe their behavior, not their identity.

Maybe you have procrastinated in the past. And maybe you still are. But that doesn't mean you will *always* procrastinate, forever and ever. Instead of thinking of yourself and telling yourself that you are a die-hard procrastinator, it's more helpful to say something like, "Yes, sometimes I procrastinate, *and* I'm learning how to better use my time."

Whenever I bring up procrastination in casual conversations, people usually half-way smile, roll their eyes, and say something like, "Oh, that's me." However, they only say that after I mention it first. We all do it. In fact, studies show that 95 percent of us admit that we procrastinate. But it's like this big secret that nobody talks about. All too often, procrastinators get used to shoving their procrastination into the back of their minds and hope it won't interfere with their goals *too* much. Sometimes they make a joke about it or try to pass it off with some lighthearted comment. They don't talk about it because it makes them feel bad and they don't know how to stop. But not talking about it makes it harder to solve the problem, so you're more likely to stay stuck. **Ignoring this particular problem doesn't make it go away.**

Once you understand what's going on inside your mind when you procrastinate, it becomes much easier to break your procrastination habits. And if you need any more incentive to figure out your own issues, here's what studies have shown:

Non-procrastinators are happier, healthier, and wealthier.

Yes, that is an extraordinary statement. Can you imagine what it would be like to live your life as a non-procrastinator? You can be one of them. My intention in writing this book is that you will hang onto your hope and be open to what this book has to offer. More happiness, health, and wealth might be right around your next corner.

Here's an example. One of my coaching clients, Alex, contacted me for help with writing a book. Alex knew he had a story to tell and important information to share, but he had been procrastinating for several years on getting started. Alex planned to start a coaching and consulting business focused on leadership, and he wanted a book as a calling card, something to help establish his credibility and expertise.

I taught Alex a number of the techniques I include in this book. Even with a demanding job, and with a wife and two kids, Alex managed to complete about a third of his book after five months of our working together. With the habits he had developed, he felt he could continue without our coaching and finish the book on his own. Alex was willing to experiment with new techniques until he found what worked for him. He deserves lots of credit for his quick turnaround and rapid progress. He was no longer willing to put his dream on hold, and he made a commitment to make that happen.

How this Book Can Help You

We live in an intense and challenging world. So many aspects of our lives are changing daily that it's sometimes hard to keep up. Many people feel they are working harder and faster to get things done, but they can't seem to make much progress. Add into that mix all our digital distractions— social media, texts, emails, online games and movies, nonstop news—and it's a wonder we get anything done at all.

I know you are probably beyond busy, and even carving out the time to read this book may feel like a stretch. But please keep going. The tips and tools will help you bypass the distractions and zero in on your most important goals, the priorities that matter most to you. You will learn how to focus on achieving the goals you already have on your to-do lists, only do them in different ways. Except for the time it takes to do the reading and the activities, you won't be adding anything new to what you need to get done. You'll just experiment with different ways to actually accomplish your goals—without the internal battle of fighting with yourself all along the way. In the long run, overcoming procrastination will save you incredible amounts of time and energy. And even though change is often difficult, it's not nearly as hard as driving with the brakes on and living the way you may be living right now.

The following chapters describe more fully the Inner Game of procrastination and give you lots of strategies to stop the internal conflicts and win the game. These ten chapters can change your life in big and small ways—if you put in the effort to change. Otherwise, this book will become like probably lots of other self-help books you've read: interesting and insightful, but not life changing. Here's how mentor and best-selling author John Assaraf describes it:

If you're interested, you'll do what's convenient. If you're committed, you'll do what it takes.

What it takes to change life-long patterns of procrastination is to release the subconscious inner blocks that may have been holding you back or find ways to work around them. Outsmart your limitations. Find a different route to the goal. You're now reading a book that can help you do that. My hope for you is that right this minute, you will make a *commitment* to do the activities that are recommended, for your own sake, for the sake of your family, friends, and coworkers, and for the sake of everyone else who will benefit when you embrace your power.

Look at it this way. You can read a book about dancing, or you can get up on your feet, go out on the dance floor, and actually learn the steps. Overcoming procrastination is about learning new skills for how to first control your thoughts, and then control your behavior. The only way you get good at it is to experiment with different strategies until you get it right. Until you find the techniques and tools that work for you. Until you find the right dance steps and practice those until they are automatic. The time it takes to learn them is relatively short. **It doesn't take that long.** Plus, you get to enjoy the learning itself, finally accomplish your goals, and feel good along the way.

You might be wondering how "working" on goals that you've been putting off for months or years could feel good. But here's the deal. Part of our survival instinct as humans is to constantly learn and grow. It's built into our DNA to perpetuate our human species. In order to ensure constant growth, Mother Nature set it up so that when we're in the process of learning and growing, it triggers a powerful chemical in the brain called **dopamine**. Dopamine makes you feel energized, excited, and happy. It motivates you to work toward future goals, because you anticipate that your success will make you feel good. Any progress you make toward those goals releases even more of this feel-good neurotransmitter. Once you accomplish your goals, dopamine is what causes you to feel high.

We all crave dopamine, almost all the time. Usually without knowing it, every day, we go around looking for ways to trigger the release of dopamine, often by pursuing goals we think will provide that reward. These goals include meeting our basic survival needs like finding food and making money. Additional activities that provide a dopamine reward include exercising, listening to music, watching television, having sex, or going onto the internet. Plus, people often seek the feel-good rewards of dopamine through drugs (including caffeine, alcohol, nicotine, and marijuana) and through certain foods (like sugar and junk food). We are constantly trying to feel good and avoid feeling bad. These kinds of activities and substances can help us do both.

Dopamine is so effective at motivating behavior that it fuels every kind of addiction there is. That's because once we find something that makes us feel good, we crave more of the dopamine it provides, so we do more of that activity. However, dopamine can be used to reward both healthy and unhealthy behavior. As a procrastinator, you can learn to switch around the rewards and let your brain reward you with dopamine when you move out of procrastination and into action. Then it becomes extra energy, a physical and emotional boost that helps you feel happy and motivated to keep going with your goals. What a welcome surprise!

Not only that, but when you master skills to overcome procrastination *while* working on your goals, **you get a double dose of dopamine**. You get to feel good for the progress you make on the goals you have been avoiding. *And* you get a dopamine reward for the progress you make as you learn new skills that keep you from procrastinating in the first place. Dopamine is the reason why success breeds success. It is why successful people seem to gain momentum and go faster and further. Even if their goals involve hard work and frustrations and setbacks, dopamine makes the learning itself feel good all along the way. You can learn how to do the same thing.

There is a great book title by Valorie Kondos Field called *Life is Short: Don't Wait to Dance*. The title rings true because life *is* short. Especially as we get older, time seems to accelerate and go by faster and faster. Time doesn't wait for anyone. It just keeps marching forward whether we're taking advantage of it or not. Which is another way of considering the question,

If not now, when?

When you look back at your life five years from now, where will you be? Will you be where you want to be? Will you have the job, the money, the house, the car, the loving relationships, the fitness and health, and the peace and happiness you want? Or will your life be pretty much the way it is now?

And *who* will you be? Will you be basically the same person you are today? Still procrastinating, still sitting on the sidelines, still knowing that you have all kinds of potential that is waiting for you to tap into? Or will you look back and be unbelievably grateful that you faced your procrastination head-on, decided to try some new techniques, and found what works for you? That you are now over-the-moon thrilled with your new life and the new you?

When people get stuck, they often try even harder by using the same techniques that haven't worked in the past. They don't want to give up, and they think that by using the same techniques just a little longer, they will eventually succeed. Sometimes that is absolutely true. But in this case, if you keep doing what you've been doing, it's almost impossible not to get the same results you've always gotten. **With procrastination, if you want things you've never had, you need to do things you've never done**. It's time to find a different way of approaching your procrastination and commit to that for long enough to get the results you want.

The activities I recommend throughout this book will help you take immediate action on your goals, including the ones you're stuck on right now. Most of the activities have successfully been used with millions of people around the world after they learned them from the coaches and mentors I have learned from. I combined what I've found to be the most effective of their techniques. I added some of my own strategies based on my education, personal experiences, and what I've learned from my university students and coaching clients. I also included new discoveries in coaching, psychology, and brain research. My hope in writing this book is that the combination of material and techniques I have included, the ways I describe them, and the activities I suggest will help you become the non-procrastinator who already lives inside of you—regardless of where you're starting from.

Here's the Plan for Your Success

You may have read other books on procrastination or time management that included helpful information but didn't work for you. Maybe you learned a few good tips, but basically you continued to do what you had always done. If you are like lots of other people, you have gotten your hopes up that you've finally found the answer, only to feel disappointed once again, almost to the point of giving up. And now you're skeptical about any books or programs that tell you changing bad habits is easy.

I've been down that road more times than I can count. I read dozens of books on time management and procrastination during my many years of teaching those classes to college students. Did all of that information help me personally stop procrastinating? Some of it did. But only when it came to doing things I already felt comfortable with. When it came to doing the scary things that flew in the face of some of my strongest subconscious beliefs, I needed much more than information about time management to change my behavior. I needed to transform the limiting beliefs that were underneath my procrastination to finally break free.

I've written this book with all of that in mind. First, I'll help you understand the reasons you procrastinate, which is essential to get past those. In the next chapter, we will look at the parts of the brain that stop you from doing what you say you want to do. Once you see exactly why you have gotten stuck with certain goals, it can help you be more forgiving and compassionate with yourself. Like those *aha* moments when you finally get it and say, "Oh, no wonder!"

Next, I will teach you a simple four-step technique to let go of the beliefs that are holding you back. What is so astounding about this technique, is that **you don't have to know what your limiting beliefs are.** You can learn to release the internal blocks they are causing, which then allows you to move forward. In all my decades of studying psychology, personal growth, and healing, and in all my searches for ways to help people get unstuck, I have never found a technique that is this simple and this fast. In fact, people who learn it often turn right around and teach it to their children.

After you learn how to release your internal blocks, you're ready to set clear goals, change your procrastination habits, and make better use of your time. New research on how to develop healthy habits is especially exciting. We now know the fastest and easiest ways to change daily habits, and those daily habits are what determine where we go in the future. You will learn how to make small shifts in your habits that eventually lead you to your goals. Instead of trying to find more time or add more habits into your day, you can replace your current habits with habits that empower you. **Once you learn how to create new habits, your life will never be the same.**

Procrastination can be particularly common in certain settings, like at work and in college. The amount of time and money lost by businesses due to procrastination is staggering. It is costing businesses countless work hours and billions of dollars. And it's getting worse. Much worse. College students live in a world of nonstop distractions that make it difficult to stay focused on their studies. Research shows that their procrastination results in lower grades, health problems, and self-confidence issues.

The techniques I describe in the following chapters work in all environments, whether you're struggling to keep up at work, or you're a student failing your classes, or an overwhelmed parent, an ambitious entrepreneur, or you're stuck in limbo in your life, believing that you're doomed to procrastinate forever. For example, you may be surprised—and relieved—to find out just how much your online screen time is contributing to your procrastination and how some simple changes can quickly turn things around.

Throughout this book, I include research on the impact technology is having on our brains and how spending hours on the internet every day (like we all do) prevents us from focusing on what is important in our lives. Do you spend too much time on your phone? If your answer is "Yes," then if you get nothing more out of this book than a better balance between the time you spend on digital distractions and the time you spend focused on your most important goals, reading this book will probably be worth it. Because so many people procrastinate by going online—then get hooked on various internet platforms like social media and video games— I've included a chapter on internet addiction and suggestions on how to overcome it (see Chapter Eight).

How to Read This Book

I encourage you to read this book from front to back. This will give you the order of information you need to be most successful in using the techniques. As you read, I suggest you highlight the sections of the book that seem the most important to you. Dog-ear the pages. Take notes. Write in the margins. Getting physically involved with the material will make it stick better in your brain. Re-reading key sections will also help you remember what's important.

However, reading and understanding will only go so far in helping you overcome deep-seated habits of procrastination. Often, **insight is not enough**. That's why throughout the book, I include activities that I enthusiastically encourage you to do. These activities will help you apply the material to your own life. They will teach you new skills and habits so you can stop wasting time and start being more productive.

Some of these activities involve writing. I suggest that you keep all your writing in one place. Some people like to use a notebook or journal. They have found that writing in longhand makes their writing a deeper experience and helps them learn better. Some people like to use their phone or computer for their writing. If that's what you prefer, there are lots of journal apps that you can download for free, or you can simply use a folder to save all your responses. Especially when you start to experiment with different strategies, it will be helpful to review what you tried before and whether it worked. Having all your writing in one place will make it easier to review later on, and there's not enough space to write all your responses in this book. Also, if you do the activities along with one or more other people who are reading this book, and if you talk about what you're learning, you will increase your chances for success even more.

How much you get out of the activities depends on how much you put into them. Just like with physical exercise, the effort you put in determines the results you get back. As author and motivational speaker Jim Rohn said, "You can't hire someone else to do your push-ups for you." This same principle applies to anything in life. If you want to learn how to play the piano, you have to sit down and practice. If you want to get better at speaking Spanish, you need to put in the time to improve.

If you are not where you want to be, at some point you will need to commit to change. This is where your past failures and frustrations can become a gift. They can get you to a place where you say, "Enough is enough. I'm ready to do whatever it takes to get past the procrastination that has already cost me too much in my life." My hope is that making that commitment will lead you to a life where you thrive as your brightest best self, as the person you were made to be, doing what you came here to do. No procrastinating. No holding back.

I have poured everything I know into this book to help you be successful with your goals, whatever those might be. I want that success to start right here, right now, with your commitment to do your part. Will you run into challenges along the way? Of course. Will you get frustrated and want to quit? Maybe. Will you get impatient that the strategies aren't working fast enough? Possibly. Significant changes in your behavior usually take consistent effort over time.

As the saying goes, "Old habits die hard." All of that is true *and* . . . there are easier ways and there are harder ways to make the changes you want in your life. I have written this book to make your journey to success as easy and as fast as possible. In the next chapter we will explore some of the obstacles that may be in your way and how to move beyond them. But before we move on, I want you to get a clear picture of the outcomes you want to achieve.

Ask Yourself, "Why Am I Reading This Book?"

It probably goes without saying that you are reading this book because you want to stop procrastinating. Right? But "to stop procrastinating" is a vague goal that can mean different things to different people. As we will cover in Chapter Six on goal setting, when you set specific goals and fill in the details on what that will mean to you, those goals become more motivating and easier to achieve. You know exactly where you are headed, and you will know exactly when you get there.

As you will see throughout this book, your hidden power to stop procrastinating is your knowledge of why you do it, your awareness of when it happens, and your ability to do something productive instead. When I wrote this book, I had a mission or purpose in mind for everyone who read it. I knew what I wanted readers to achieve:

By the end of this book, you will understand why you procrastinate, master new skills to stop procrastinating, become more productive in general, and achieve at least one short-term goal that is important to you.

When you achieve that one important goal, it will indicate that you have accomplished the other parts of this mission, at least enough to get you moving toward your goals instead of away from them. After you finish reading the book, you will need to keep practicing. But **the skills you will develop along the way are skills you can use for the rest of your life.**

Right now, identify one goal you want to achieve by the time you finish reading this book. Make sure it is realistic and doable in only a few weeks. If you want to choose a long-term goal to work on, then focus on completing one or more short-term goals that will help you achieve your long-term goal. Once you decide on a goal, then take the next few minutes and answer the following questions. These questions come from sport psychology and are used to help athletes achieve the results they want. They can help anyone else who wants to use them, including you, because they're based on brain research.

Study after study has shown that your mind doesn't know the difference between imagining something in the future and actually experiencing it as a reality in your life right now. That's why this type of success imagery is so effective with professional athletes. Anticipating future success is part of what drives them to work for years to finally make it to first place or to win that prized gold medal. It helps them tap into dopamine and gives them an energy boost to keep going. Imagining how phenomenal their success will feel means they get more good feelings and feel even better each step along the way.

You can use this same type of imagery to help you keep going until you win your equivalent of the gold. Writing down your goals makes you much more likely to achieve them. Write down the goal you want to achieve by the time you've finished reading this book. Also write down the images you get in your mind as you answer the following questions. Describe what you want in the present tense, as if it is has already come true and is already happening.

1. **What will it _look_ like when you achieve your goal?** In your mind, decide on a picture of your ultimate success. Just like in running a race, where crossing the finish line—with your hands held high—symbolizes success, you can create a picture in your mind that is your equivalent of crossing the finish line when you complete your goal.

   When I first started writing this book, I wanted a picture in my head of what success would look like. I designed a book cover that might be something like my published book, and I printed that design on a piece of paper. I stuck the paper on my refrigerator, and it stayed there until this book came out. It became my symbol of success for completing the book. Every day it reminded me of what I was working toward.

You can do something similar with your goal. Decide on a picture of what that will look like. Then get a real picture or an object that represents your ultimate success and keep it someplace where you will see it often.

2. **What will it _sound_ like when you achieve your goal?** Take a moment right now to imagine that when you finish reading this book, you have been 100 percent successful in reaching your goal. What does that sound like?

What are the sounds you hear *outside* of yourself, the ones coming from your environment? Maybe you can hear people congratulating you on your achievement. Perhaps you hear people thanking you for doing something you have been putting off. Or maybe you hear the happy sounds of your children's voices if your goal is to spend less time on your phone and more time with them.

What are the sounds you hear *inside* of yourself when you have completed your goal with 100 percent success? What are the kinds of things you might be saying to yourself? Maybe your self-talk will be something like, "Wow. I did it!" Or "I'm so glad I hung in there until I achieved my goal." What do you imagine you might say to yourself? Write down a few examples of what you might say to yourself when you cross over the finish line of what success means to you.

3. **What will it _feel_ like when you get the results you want?** Take another moment to imagine that you have been completely successful with your goal. Imagine what that will feel like. Let yourself feel those emotions right now as you anticipate your success.

Maybe you feel over-the-top happy, knowing your happiness is well deserved and that it's a reason to celebrate. Or maybe you feel a healthy sense of pride and satisfaction that comes from doing your part and hanging in there until you get the results you want. Whatever you imagine you might feel when you symbolically win your race, let yourself feel it now.

This imagery is most effective when you imagine feeling the good feelings your success will bring for about thirty seconds. At first, this may seem like a long time. But with practice, you'll start to enjoy it. I suggest thirty seconds because as we will cover in Chapter Seven, **by using your emotions, you can learn something new and change your behavior faster than with any other techniques**.

After you do this imagery, then say to yourself, "This or something better." Often, what we achieve is even better than what we imagined, so it's important to allow for this possibility. To make this imagery even more powerful, see, hear, and feel your success at least weekly—and better yet daily—until you reach your finish line. One of the best times to do this imagery is right before you go to sleep. Your subconscious mind can then focus on the outcomes you want all during the night. When you get up the next morning, your brain is already programmed to succeed.

Please note that some people don't actually see pictures in their heads when they do this type of imagery, and they may have difficulty hearing sounds or feeling emotions. If you're one of them, that's okay. You can still benefit from trying it out, so keep practicing.

I've been doing this imagery for more than twenty years with my individual clients, with students in my classes, and with people in my trainings and talks. When I have a chance to get feedback from them after they have tried it on their own, they usually tell me they're amazed at how easy it was to succeed at their goals. That's because in their minds, they had already practiced completing their goals. Perfectly.

As we end the second chapter of this book, I want to congratulate you on reading this far. Less than ten percent of people who buy a book read past the first chapter, so you are already ahead of the curve. Good for you!

Chapter 2 Highlights

At the end of each chapter, I will include a section called Highlights. This section will list some of the most important points from that chapter to help you better understand procrastination. If you know the tactics of your Inner Game and Outer Game opponents and how they operate, it's easier to plan strategies to outsmart your opponents and win the game. You will also find several recommended activities or **action steps** that were described in the chapter and that I wholeheartedly encourage you to do.

1. The good news is that procrastination is learned. You weren't born a procrastinator. You learned to procrastinate, and you can learn to

replace it with productive behaviors instead.

2. The Inner Game of procrastination is what goes on in your head that keeps you from taking action on your plans. Resolving the conflicts created by your subconscious mind means you can start getting things done and keep going. The results are usually sustainable.

3. Many experts agree that at least 80 percent of all the obstacles we face in life have to do with the Inner Game. Outer Game obstacles are the ones in our environment (like time and money), and they comprise no more than 20 percent of what gets in the way of our success.

4. Once you learn how win the Inner Game of procrastination, you can use the same techniques to get past the obstacles in every other area of your life where you have internal blocks. These skills can change the quality of your life from here on out.

5. You can learn how to release your brain's feel-good hormone called dopamine when you stop procrastinating and move into action.

6. When compared to people who procrastinate, non-procrastinators are happier, healthier, and wealthier. You can be among them.

Action Steps

The action steps that I suggest at the end of each chapter can help you gradually become a happy and productive non-procrastinator. Some people get hung up on wanting to do these activities perfectly. If they can't be perfect, then they don't do them at all. Perfectionism can be a trap that keeps you stuck. The goal here is to take **imperfect action**. Don't wait for that illusive moment when you think you can do them exactly right. You don't need for these steps to be perfect. What's important is to have them *done*.

1. Guilt doesn't help. Instead of guilt tripping yourself when you procrastinate, use self-compassion and forgiveness. That will help you make more progress, faster. And besides, it's really *not* your fault.

2. Taking on procrastination as part of your identity cements it into your brain and makes it harder to change. Rather than telling yourself or others, "I'm a procrastinator," instead say, "Sometimes I procrastinate, *and* I'm learning how to use my time in better ways."

3. Imagine what it will be like in a few short weeks when you have finished reading this book. Imagine that you have been 100 percent

successful in achieving at least one goal that is important to you. See, hear, and feel your success. Do this often. Your brain will release dopamine as if you're already there.

Chapter 3

Why Do We Procrastinate?

Procrastination can be seen in every culture, and it can invade every aspect of our lives. In his book *The Procrastination Equation*, researcher Piers Steel says that procrastination

> *". . . is about every promise you made to yourself but broke. It is about every goal you set but let slide, never finding the motivation. It is about diets postponed, late-night scrambles to finish project . . . It is about that menacing cloud of uncompleted chores, from the late bill payments to the clutter that fills your home. It is about that doctor's appointment you have been putting off and the finances still in disarray. It is about dawdling, delay, opportunity lost, and more. Much more."*

Yes, procrastination is a pervasive, universal problem, so common that many people think it is normal. I was and wasn't surprised to learn that at any given time, "To stop procrastinating" is among the top reported goals—in the *world*. That's a lot of procrastinators. You're definitely not alone in your struggles to overcome it. In this chapter we will look at why so many of us stall, shoot ourselves in the foot, and sabotage the very goals we say we want to achieve.

It pays to know why. It is worth taking a little time to understand it. That's because studies show that people who understand the reasons they procrastinate are more successful in overcoming it. Besides, if you're like most chronic procrastinators, you have already tried the standard Outer Game advice for procrastinators, like time management and goal setting tips, and those alone didn't work, or at least not for long. Through your best intentions, you jumped right into trying to change your behavior, but the underlying issues never got resolved, and pretty soon, you fell right back into your old habits. Or maybe you had some success, but not a lot.

My goal is to help you change your behavior for the long haul. In this book, we're going for sustainable success, not temporary fixes. For you to first identify the causes of your procrastination—and based on those—*then* change your behavior. So let's explore the parts of your brain that are responsible for your repeated delays. Then you will know why the strategies and brain hacks throughout the rest of this book work, and you can more easily apply them in your own life for more permanent, long-term results.

We all like to think of ourselves as intelligent human beings who make conscious decisions about what we do and how we direct the course of our lives. But the truth is that about 95 percent of how we live our lives is directed by the subconscious mind, which is outside of our conscious awareness. The conscious mind and the subconscious mind are often in conflict, especially when you want to accomplish a goal that will take you to a new and improved place in your life. If it is some place better and new (like every one of your self-improvement goals), your subconscious mind will often see it as "not normal" and may try to sabotage your efforts. And if that goal also contradicts your limiting beliefs? Oh, boy. Your efforts to reach your goal will usually either be painfully slow or will come to a complete stop.

You can sometimes catch a glimpse of these conflicts in your mind if you have ever noticed that you were arguing with yourself. Not out loud, but in your head. It's like there are two different people or parts inside of you, with two distinct voices. Your internal conversation might go something like this:

Part 1: "You need to get that done."
Part 2: "I know, but I don't feel like it right now."

Part 1: "It's due in two days. It's a big project, and it's important."
Part 2: "I know. I can do it later. Besides, it won't take that long."

Part 1: "It's stressing you out to keep putting it off."
Part 2: "I deserve a short break. I'll just check Facebook really fast. Then I'll get started."

Part 1: (Sometime later) "You've been on Facebook for over an hour. You're running out of time for your project! What's wrong with you?"
Part 2: "It's okay. I can stay up late tonight and work on it. Besides, I

work well under pressure."

And so, you put it off again. You stay stuck in your avoidance and the project gets shelved once more. Your procrastination just won that round of the Inner Game. **Usually, the voice that has the last word wins**. If you don't come up with a rebuttal, the game is over. As you will learn, it's extremely helpful to focus on the conversation between the two parts of yourself and become more aware of that internal dialog. Then you can learn to change your self-talk, which makes it possible to change your behavior.

This example demonstrates several characteristics about procrastinators that keep them stuck. They often falsely believe they do their best work when under pressure. It's probably more accurate to say they finally get started when they're smack-dab up against a deadline and are so panicked that their adrenaline level is sky high.

Procrastinators are also notorious for doing two things: they *overestimate* the time remaining to complete a goal; they also *underestimate* the amount of time it will take to complete it. In other words, they often think they have more time to complete a goal than they actually have. They also tend to think they can complete a goal in less time than it will actually take. In general, they wait until the last minute, and depending on the kind of task it is, they don't leave themselves enough time to do quality work, much less sleep on the work they have completed, mull it over, and look for ways to make it better. They rush to finish, and even if they meet their deadline, they end up stressed and disappointed with themselves. And then they turn right around and do it again, like they didn't learn a thing from their experience. But as long as your subconscious inner opponents remain hidden in the dark shadows of your brain, then just like a knee-jerk reaction, they will "make" you procrastinate over and over again. It's time to get out your flashlight, shine a light into that darkness, and increase your odds of winning the Inner Game.

What is Procrastination?

To better understand the conflicts in your mind, it helps to first define procrastination. What exactly are we talking about? **Procrastination is needless delay.** You have time to get something done, or you could make the time, but you don't. Whether you are consciously aware of it or not, you wait to act on a goal and sabotage your efforts to achieve it. This self-defeating habit doesn't make logical sense until you put it in context. And here's the deal.

One of the most basic human instincts is that we seek pleasure and avoid pain. It's another survival mechanism built into our DNA. When we procrastinate, we usually choose some kind of short-term pleasure in order to avoid short-term emotional discomfort, because discomfort registers in our brains as a form of pain.

Most of the time, the uncomfortable feelings don't come from the task itself. In fact, the vast majority of the time, **it isn't the task you are avoiding, it's the emotions that go along with it.** Just thinking about doing the task can make you feel stressed, overwhelmed, or anxious. This is a huge part of procrastination. You don't want to feel stressed out in the moment, so you put something off and end up feeling worse later on. Usually, it is because you simply don't know how else to deal with those unpleasant feelings or emotions, and you procrastinate instead. So basically, **procrastination is a coping strategy to avoid uncomfortable emotions.**

Because of your hardwired survival instincts, it's normal to want to avoid things that make you feel uncomfortable. But when hesitation and delays become a pattern in your life, those will inevitably lead to regret. You will miss out on opportunities and may feel like life is passing you by. Because it is.

Knowing the definition of procrastination makes this another one of those situations where you need to cut yourself some slack. Very, very few people are taught healthy ways to deal with any uncomfortable emotions— even common ones like sadness and disappointment—much less the ones that often show up when we procrastinate (like intense fear, dread, shame, and helplessness). What do we do instead? We avoid feeling those feelings, which often means we avoid the tasks that trigger those feelings. And not only do we avoid unpleasant feelings, when we procrastinate, we usually do something else that makes us feel good, at least in that moment. We follow the basic programming of our DNA to avoid pain and seek pleasure.

Based on the definition of procrastination, you might be wondering if all your gyrations and delay tactics with procrastination mostly boil down to avoiding uncomfortable emotions and trying to feel good. You probably already know that you avoid doing things that make you feel bad. But are you stalling with feel-good activities instead? Let's test it out. Right now, ask yourself this question:

What do you do to avoid what you should be doing?

In other words, what are your **avoidance activities**? Most of us have several, but pick the one you do the most often. For example, do you check social media, email or text, binge on Netflix, watch YouTube videos, play online games, turn on the TV, eat when you're not hungry, take a nap, catch up on the news? What is your main go-to avoidance activity, the one you use the most?

Now think back on a time when you either consciously chose to do that avoidance activity, or you unconsciously just started doing it. Remember how it made you feel. Chances are high that your avoidance activity somehow makes you feel good. If nothing else, it's a great escape. It gets you away from the bad feelings of facing something you don't want to do. It also helps you avoid the guilt of not doing what you should be doing. As we will discuss more later on, going online almost always rewards us with dopamine, so most digital activities will give you an immediate feeling of excitement and pleasure.

When I ask the people in my workshops about their avoidance activities, most say they go online. Some people eat, clean, sleep, read, shop, or find someone to talk to. But every example of an avoidance activity that people have mentioned to me has some kind of feel-good component. Procrastination gets us hooked because it's a double whammy: you get to avoid doing something that makes you feel bad, and you get to do something else that makes you feel good, at least in the short run. No wonder procrastination can become such a strong habit.

But our avoidance activities also have an emotional downside. The whole time you're engaged in your avoidance activities, somewhere in the back of your mind, you know you should be doing something else. Just under the surface of your feel-good escape, you probably feel a pinch of guilt. You know you haven't earned your fun time, and you know you will pay a price for your delays in the long run. It's hard to truly enjoy avoidance activities because you know you're wasting time, so they end up being your guilty pleasures.

Awareness is the key here. From now on, whenever you find yourself engaged in your favorite avoidance activity, simply ask yourself, "Am I procrastinating?" Maybe you are, maybe you're not. However, if you identify what you do to let yourself off the hook, you can start to become more consciously aware of your pattern of procrastination—as you are doing it. Noticing when you procrastinate gives you an advantage point, a slight edge in eventually winning the Inner Game, because awareness is the first step in breaking bad habits and changing your behavior.

Can procrastination ever be a good thing? Yes. On relatively rare occasions, it can be better to postpone something and do it later. We will discuss those situations later on. Right now though, let's focus on when your delays are self-defeating. How can you tell the difference between justifiable and self-defeating procrastination? When you are trying to convince yourself that your stalling is a good thing, there will always be an emotional twinge. Somewhere inside, you will feel a pang of guilt or regret, almost like you already know that somewhere down the road, you'll wish you had gotten something done sooner rather than later. When you are in doubt about whether to wait, ask yourself this question: "Will I regret this?" It doesn't help to try to fool yourself, so be as honest as you can be when you answer. Even if you know in advance you will regret your procrastination, you may still decide to wait.

Avoidance Activities Can Change Over Time

I spent so many years trying to overcome my procrastination that now I can see how my avoidance activities changed over time. I used to stall by doing some low priority task instead of what I needed to do. I would clean my house or do some kind of busywork like responding to emails or paying bills. I might not have been working on my top priority, but at least I was getting something done. This is sometimes called **productive procrastination,** where you put off the thing you most need to do by doing something else that isn't as urgent.

Sometimes I would watch television, but then I got rid of my TV, which was one of the best things I've ever done for myself. Watching television leaves me feeling passive and dull, and afterward, it's hard for me to get motivated to do anything productive. I remember having a brief panic attack when I carried my TV out of my living room and put it in my car to take to the recycler. And I remember thinking *What am I going to do when I feel anxious?* However, I'm convinced that it would have been harder to write my first book and this book if my TV had been such a convenient distraction.

But I quickly learned how to substitute what I was getting from watching television with going online. And I don't just mean the information and programs. I noticed that when I was avoiding something I needed to get done, or when I needed a break, or when I was bored, or when I felt upset, I would suddenly become a news junkie and surf the internet for what could become several hours. Digital distraction became my go-to avoidance activity, and there was nothing productive about it.

I was shocked to realize how easy it was to lose track of time when I was online. Not only that, but I didn't seem to get tired while I was doing it, even if I was sitting all slumped over with terrible posture and hardly breathing. After I learned about dopamine, I realized I was probably on a dopamine high. But just like when I would watch television, long periods of time on the internet left me feeling passive, a little spacey, and definitely not in the mood to do anything that required focus or concentration. As you will learn later, my reactions make complete sense based on how our brains work.

How Your Subconscious Mind Sabotages Your Success

Have you ever looked at successful people and wondered why it seems so easy for them? What their secret is? Why they seem to be living their dreams, and yet you keep procrastinating on even getting to first base? Why have you longed for success for years, probably worked hard to make it happen, and yet you're still struggling to get the income you want, a more satisfying career, a healthier lifestyle, or the soul mate you've been searching for? And how do successful people breeze past the distractions that repeatedly trip you up and waste your time? Our subconscious minds have the answers.

We're born into this world like little psychic sponges. Up until around the age of six, our subconscious minds soak up everything around us. Everything. Mostly from our parents and other family members, but also from friends, caregivers, teachers, situations in our environment, and the culture at the time. Whether it's through actual words, watching other people's behavior, innuendos like sighs, subtle laughs, gestures, or facial expressions, it all goes straight into the subconscious. We're able to absorb enormous amounts of information because our young brains don't have the ability to filter or judge information as true or false. Whatever we learn becomes The Truth.

For example, if your parents fought a lot, you may have learned that

Relationships are painful. If your father lost his job when you were four, you may have learned that *Money is scarce and hard to get.* If your older brother picked on you and told you that you were stupid, you probably grew up believing *I'm stupid.* These are examples of limiting beliefs.

Many therapists report that the most common limiting belief they see is *I'm not good enough.* That belief has several variations, including *I don't do enough, I'm not deserving,* and *I'm not capable.* Specific examples include *I'm not smart enough, I'm not attractive enough, I'm too old/young,* and *I'm not the kind of person who could do something like that.* Often these beliefs live below your level of conscious awareness. But if you ask yourself, "Why can't I do X?" sometimes they will pop into your mind.

In contrast, if you looked around and saw that all the people in your family were successful, you probably believe that *I can be successful.* If your parents were efficient and productive, you may have learned *It's easy to get things done on time.* If you were treated with love and respect, most likely you grew up believing that *I'm worthy of love and respect.* These empowering beliefs are truly a gift. Beliefs you learn about yourself, about your identity and who you are as a person, are the basis for your self-esteem and have the greatest influence over your life.

Around the age of seven, our brains change and are no longer so open and receptive to new learning. We start to develop more conscious awareness, including filters and the ability to judge things as true or false. But what we learned before this time remains in our subconscious minds like the software program we forgot we installed on our computer. This program goes on autopilot and continues to control our thoughts, beliefs, and behaviors—for the rest of our lives—unless we go back and reprogram it later on. Not many people ever do this, except when they get into therapy or rehab or go through some belief-changing experience.

That means that most older children, adolescents, and adults are responding to situations from the beliefs of a six-year-old. Yikes! No wonder some full-grown adults act so childish at times. They may make you feel frustrated and angry. They may make you wonder why in the world anyone would think or act that way. But from a brain development standpoint, more often than not, they can't help it. They are simply acting out of their subconscious programming. They learned it from their parents, who learned it from their parents, and on up the line. It got passed down through generations like surnames in a family tree.

As little seven-year-olds, we enter the world pre-programmed with beliefs about ourselves, relationships, money, politics, religion, you name it, and those beliefs can either be limiting or empowering. Successful people usually got a generous dose of empowering beliefs. Either that, or they made a decision that they would not repeat the negative patterns in their family, changed their beliefs, and deliberately set out to create a positive, empowering life for themselves. You will also sometimes see this happen when people become parents, and they work hard not to treat their children the way they were treated, not to teach them what they themselves were taught.

Our beliefs create our reality. They provide the blueprint for our lives, which means they become self-fulfilling prophecies, whether we like it or not. No matter how much you might want to achieve a certain goal, no matter how many books you read or how many times or ways you try to make it happen, your beliefs will almost always determine the outcome and whether you succeed. Maybe you can muscle your way through with enormous amounts of time and effort. But even if you succeed, chances are good that you won't enjoy your success, or you will unconsciously find a way to blow it.

According to some reports, around 70 percent of the people who win the lottery go bankrupt in five years. Their subconscious beliefs don't change when they win, and they eventually return to a life that is consistent with their limiting beliefs about money. In his classic book *The Biology of Belief*, biologist Bruce Lipton states, "The biggest impediment to realizing the successes of which we dream are the limitations programmed into the subconscious." Oprah Winfrey said it like this,

You don't get what you wish for. You get what you believe.

The tough thing about these deep-seated beliefs is that as an adult, you usually are not consciously aware of them. Your beliefs are operating in the background, controlling your every thought, your every move, but **you usually don't know that**. Maybe you've figured out some of your limiting beliefs, but the ones that keep stopping you in your tracks often remain silent and invisible. That's why certain goals can be so, *so* difficult to achieve.

Your Subconscious Mind Wants to Keep You Safe

As we just covered, the subconscious mind is responsible for the tremendous amount of learning required for babies to get socialized into their families by the time they are seven. However, the countless number of beliefs they learn usually aren't their beliefs. Most of those beliefs have been passed down through the generations and may have absolutely nothing to do with who those little babies are with all their uniqueness and potential. But the babies grow into children who must abide by those beliefs—some of which are false beliefs—or else they are likely to get in trouble.

It is important to understand that the subconscious mind absorbs these beliefs in order **to keep you safe**. Physically safe. Emotionally safe. And mentally safe enough that you can learn, grow, and hopefully thrive. In general, the more you follow your family's beliefs as a child, the more you stay safe and don't get in trouble. These beliefs are formed for your benefit at the time, as a survival mechanism to get you safely through your childhood years. And to help you get the love, attention, and approval of those around you, which of course, we all need.

As we grow into adolescents and adults, our situations change. We start to have more freedom and choices, and the beliefs that kept us safe as children may no longer benefit us. We can outgrow them, and they can start to hold us back. Maybe you learned that *Children should be seen and not heard.* If you decide when you're nineteen that you want to be a schoolteacher, that belief may get in your way. How can you teach if you're now shy and are supposed to be quiet? Maybe you had a parent with an addiction or a mental health issue and you learned that *My job is to take care of my parent.* Later on, you may find yourself being a codependent caregiver in your close relationships. Or maybe as a young adult you want to find your special someone and get married. But if your parents got divorced when you were young, you may believe that *Marriage doesn't last*, and now you're afraid to make commitments.

Your subconscious mind doesn't know how to evaluate what's good or bad, right or wrong about your beliefs. All it knows how to do is keep playing the same tapes, keep running the same software program that got installed when you were a child. Unless you deliberately change your beliefs, they will continue to direct your life. Sometimes life experiences can help you change them. Let's say you were taught *It's not okay to make mistakes.* And yet at times, you've made mistakes that helped you learn something valuable. If you are open to them, personal experiences can override the subconscious tapes in your mind, because they can show you that your original beliefs were false to start with.

Most parents want the world for their children. They love them with all their hearts and try in earnest to give them the best they can. When some people first discover where their limiting beliefs came from, they get angry at their parents. But blaming your parents for your limiting beliefs is like blaming someone for the color of their eyes or for the fact that they are short instead of tall. Your parents unknowingly got programmed when they were children the same way all the rest of us did. They were probably doing the best they could with what they had been taught.

We need to figure out why we procrastinate so we can get past it, but this is one of those no-fault situations. Getting caught up in a blame game simply keeps you spinning your wheels even longer. However, it sometimes seems natural to be mad at the people who taught you your limiting beliefs. Later on, I will show you techniques to release your anger if that's the case for you.

Comfort Zones

Each of us has what's called a **comfort zone**. This is what's familiar, what we're used to, our "normal," and how we have lived our lives up until now. This zone is where we have managed to stay safe enough to get to where we are today. The subconscious mind operates on the belief that anything outside your comfort zone could be life threatening. It is so intent on keeping you safe that every time you step outside your comfort zone, alarms may go off, saying "Danger. Danger!" These alarms may show up in your body as adrenaline or the increased heart rate of your fight, flight, or freeze response. When you feel your body revving up, it is usually because of emotions, such as doubt and fear. Your alarms may show up as limiting thoughts (*This isn't going to work* or *Don't do that!*). And your subconscious mind may try to keep you safe through avoidance behaviors, like when you suddenly find yourself procrastinating or you simply can't force yourself do something.

It's easy to underestimate the intensity of your internal alarm system. Sometimes the danger signals are so strong that it can feel like you will literally die if you don't pay attention to their warnings. But all of this is absolutely normal, predictable, and to be expected. Stepping out of your comfort zone can trigger your **fear of the unknown**, which is one of the strongest fears we have. Your racing heart, fears, limiting thoughts, and avoidance don't necessarily mean you need to slow down or stop moving forward. At times, yes, they may be warning you of valid safety concerns that you need to address. So always pay attention to your hesitancy and doubts. But usually they are simply telling you that you're moving out of your comfort zone and heading for something different. And "different" is required if you want something better. Your life has to change in order to improve. As author Robert Allen said,

Everything you want is just outside your comfort zone.

This quote highlights the fact that when you set new goals, try to improve your life, change for the better, or reach for that next level, your subconscious alarms may seem to scream, "No, No, NO!" It is crucial for you to understand what's going on, or else you may automatically interpret your reactions to mean there's real danger ahead. And if that happens, you are likely to retreat back into your comfort zone, where your life stays the way it always has been. You will remain stuck in your past beliefs and stuck in your life.

There are ways you can stack the odds in your favor for when you reach this tricky place between the conflicting parts of your brain. For example, if you already have empowering beliefs about yourself and your ability to take risks, it will be easier to move past your subconscious alarms and continue going forward. If your beliefs include ones like *I can be successful* and *I'll figure it out*, your beliefs will usually give you the confidence to keep going, and you will almost always find a way to accomplish what you want. We will discuss a number of techniques for getting past your comfort zone in later chapters.

I recently watched a video about a small group of young people, probably in their early to mid-twenties, who understood how comfort zones can keep our lives small and constricted. They traveled all over the world together, taking adventures that forced them out of their comfort zones and face-to-face with their fears. Jumping out of airplanes, plunging into ice water, trekking across a snow-covered mountain in the dead of winter wearing only boots, gloves, and shorts or bathing suits (yes, they actually did that and came out unscathed). Mind over matter. Blasting past their fears. These courageous souls understood the value of expanding their "normal" and not allowing their subconscious beliefs to rule their lives. I'm not suggesting that you go to extremes like they did. But don't you think it's time for you to at least take some small steps to get out of your comfort zone and into a better life?

We live most of our lives on autopilot, not consciously thinking about why we may feel unworthy, why we get into relationships with people who don't treat us with respect, or why we only make enough money to just get by. Because the limiting beliefs contained in our programming can be so detrimental to our success and happiness throughout life, the following chapters will teach you how to change your beliefs and the paralyzing hold they may have on you.

For now, just know that yes, you got programmed and yes, you can replace any limiting beliefs with empowering ones. It's not your fault that you ended up exactly where you are right now. But if you want your life to get better, it is your responsibility to change it.

The Stories We Tell

No matter where I go, I often end up talking with people about procrastination. Once while out shopping, I met an impressive young woman named Alyssa who stood right there in the middle of the store and told me her whole life story.

Alyssa said she came from a family where her father demanded unwavering obedience to whatever he said. No one dared to question him, certainly none of his four children, and not even his wife. In her early twenties, Alyssa had had enough, and she moved out to live with her boyfriend. That's when she started to realize how much she had been programmed by the beliefs in her family. She kept hearing a voice in her head that said, "You'll never be successful." She suddenly realized that was what she had heard from her father through his words, a look, a tone of voice, and through annoyed, dismissive reactions to anything she did well.

Once that door of awareness opened, Alyssa began to hear another voice in her head that was the voice of her mother. She realized she was overly critical of herself and that those critical thoughts originated from both parents. At one point, she said to me, "I sound just like my mother."

Deep inside, however, Alyssa felt determined to succeed, so she started reading self-help books, listening to podcasts, watching TED talks, and searching for any information that would help her understand what was going on. By the time she was in her mid-twenties, she had developed remarkable insight for someone her age and was starting to uncover the subconscious, limiting beliefs that had kept her life in limbo. Her motivation and courage were inspiring. Alyssa's success was almost guaranteed, because she was getting to the underlying cause of what was holding her back.

All of us have a life story. Alyssa told me hers in only a few minutes. Since you're reading this book, I assume that embedded in your life story is also a procrastination story. Do you know what your procrastination story is? The one you keep repeating in your life? What patterns keep showing up in your life because you've been a procrastinator? All you need to do is look at your life from a different perspective and ask yourself, "What is the underlying procrastination story here?"

One of the things I find so fascinating about procrastination is how our limiting beliefs can weave together into patterns that become **procrastination styles**. For example, I meet a lot of people who tell me, "I procrastinate because I'm a perfectionist." They want to do everything perfectly, and because doing anything perfectly is almost impossible, they wait to even begin. Or they never finish, because it isn't perfect. When I was counseling procrastinators, I found that many perfectionists grew up with constant criticism from those around them. Nothing they did was ever good enough, and they concluded that *I'm not good enough*. Their perfectionism was their attempt to finally be good enough, to finally do it right, to finally please the people who told them their efforts fell short, or to at least get them off their backs.

Linda Sapadin, psychologist, coach, and author, focuses her therapy practice on helping her clients progress past their procrastination blocks. Curious about why some procrastinators make significant changes in therapy while others remain stuck, Sapadin sent out a questionnaire and interviewed people from all walks of life. From that research, she found that there were six styles of procrastination. Here's a brief description of those styles. More information about these six styles can be found in Sapadin's book, *How to Beat Procrastination in the Digital Age*, and at *PsychWisdom.com*.

As you read through this list, notice any descriptions that seem true for you.

1. **Perfectionist**. Perfectionists find it tough to complete a task because they don't want to do anything that is less than a perfect job. They may be concerned about satisfying their own high standards or satisfying

the high standards their parents had for them. Their underlying limiting belief is that *I'm not good enough* or that *What I've done is not good enough.*

2. **Dreamer**. Imaginative and creative, Dreamers can come up with plenty of grand ideas for what they want in their future. But they are passive when it comes to doing the work to turn those ideas into realities. They like the thought of reaching their future goals but lack the skills to follow through and make them happen. Their underlying limiting belief is that *I have great ideas but acting on those ideas to turn them into realities is difficult for me.*

3. **Worrier**. Worriers zoom in on potential problems, using them as reasons to procrastinate. They have difficulty making decisions and are afraid of change because of all the what-ifs that might happen. They're lacking in self-confidence, don't trust themselves to be able to handle problems, and their underlying limiting belief is that *I doubt my own abilities.*

4. **Crisis Maker**. It is difficult for Crisis Makers to start a task until the last minute. The anxiety of an approaching deadline is what gives them the energy and motivation to finally get going. If they pull it off in time, they then feel like a hero. Their underlying limiting belief is that *I need a crisis to get motivated and feel alive.*

5. **Defier**. People with a Defier style will often disagree with the fact that they need to do something in the first place. If they find they have to do it, they may become resentful and angry, and then drag their feet on getting it done. Their underlying limiting belief is that *I should only have to do what I want to do.*

6. **Pleaser**. Those with a Pleaser style find it hard to say "No" to other people's requests. They often overcommit, spread themselves too thin, and end up procrastinating on things they need to do for themselves. Their underlying limiting belief is that *My self-worth depends on other people's approval.*

Do any of these sound familiar? You may relate to more than one style, but together they can help you identify your procrastination story. Alyssa didn't mention having a problem with perfectionism, but based on her impeccable appearance (clothes, hair, makeup), it might have been there. Alyssa's procrastination story can be described as simply as,

My parents constantly criticized me when I was growing up. I internalized what they said and became overly critical of myself. My father also told me I would never succeed. For many years, I believed him, and up until my twenties, I held myself back from even trying to do things that would make me look successful.

My own procrastination story is a little longer and goes like this:

With two older sisters, I was "the baby" in our family, but I didn't get spoiled the way many babies do. My parents were extraordinarily good people and good parents, and they did their best to make everything fair and equal among their three daughters. Despite their best intentions, from that I learned two limiting beliefs: Don't outshine others and Don't be too powerful. I tried hard not to look better than my sisters or any of my cousins, not to outshine anyone—or else then things wouldn't be equal. Because my sisters and cousins were older and excelled in a lot of areas I might have enjoyed (academics, sports, music, art), those became areas where I felt like I needed to hold back.

All little kids need activities where they can do well, areas where they can feel accomplished and empowered. I didn't have that. When I was in the third grade, I stumbled onto a way to feel powerful by making other people wait on me. From then on, I was often late, feeling power over others with my defiance. (the Defier style). *I was angry about having to hold back and mad about having to do things I didn't want to do. Being late became my passive-aggressive act of protest.* (Yes, that's hard to admit.)

I figured out how to overcome some of my procrastination and had a successful career, but I stayed in my safe comfort zone, only going so far, until I retired to start my own business. My career goals changed, and I wanted to help as many people as I could. Thousands, if not more. If I succeeded, it would mean outshining other family members and appearing to be too powerful. That's when I ran into a second procrastination roadblock that brought my new career to a screeching halt.

Fortunately, my story didn't end there. I realized that remnants of my limiting beliefs were still holding me back. Plus, my new career goals were way too far outside my comfort zone not to trigger a massive fear reaction. In order to get unstuck, I needed to first change my story about what my future could look like, to open my mind to the possibility that I could live a better life and a more fulfilling life than the one I had been living. If you're like I was, and procrastination still has a tight grip on you, keep reading. This next section describes how to turn your procrastination

44

story into a story of success.

How to Change Your Procrastination Story in Three Short Steps

Now it's your turn to open up to the possibility of a better life for yourself. Grab some paper or hop on your phone or computer and write down your responses in each of the following three steps. Keep your responses with the rest of the writing you're doing as you go through this book.

Step 1. Write down your procrastination story.

What is your procrastination story? Write your story as you understand it today. It may only be a few paragraphs, or longer if you want, but it can help you get some distance from your automatic, knee-jerk reactions and start to become more aware of your patterns. Here are some questions that might help you piece it together.

- When do you first remember procrastinating?
- Do you remember what happened *after* the first time you procrastinated and how that made you feel?
- What patterns do you see in your life that happen over and over because of your repeated delays?
- Do you know what limiting belief(s) might be underneath your procrastination?
- Can you see any of the six procrastination styles in your story?

Okay. Did you get your story written down? I hope so, because this is an important part of changing your mindset and overcoming the obstacles that are keeping you stuck.

Step 2. Write a happy ending to your procrastination story.

Obviously, your story is not over yet. You haven't gotten to the end. And thankfully, you can change the ending of your story to be whatever you want. Whatever you can imagine would be the best ending for you. No matter how bad your procrastination has been up until now, you get to decide the final outcome. You get to give your procrastination story a happy ending.

Alyssa's happy ending might be that,

I finally get to the bottom of why I procrastinate, change my beliefs, learn how to accomplish my goals, and enjoy a happy and successful life. This includes getting married to my boyfriend, graduating from college, and becoming a life coach where I help other people overcome their limiting beliefs.

I'm already living the happy ending to my story, which is that,

I keep searching for answers and finally figure out all the pieces of my procrastination. I say "Yes" to my new career goal and then help as many other procrastinators as I can through speaking, consulting, coaching, and publishing my book. If procrastination starts to creep back into my life, I use my tried-and-true techniques to help me stay on track. These techniques include changing my limiting beliefs and not allowing fear to stop me when I venture out of my comfort zone.

Again, it's your turn. Write a happy ending to your procrastination story. It doesn't have to be long. Sometimes just another short paragraph is enough. This will start giving your mind different ideas and instructions about your future. Write the parts that haven't happened yet in the present tense, like the two examples above.

Step 3. Be grateful for the lessons you have learned.
None of us want to look back at parts of our life that feel negative or that leave us feeling like we failed, even if it wasn't our fault. An important part of being able to create a happy ending to your procrastination story is to accept it up until now as exactly as it was, as stressful and self-sabotaging as it may have been. Your acceptance can allow you to see that part of your past in a positive way, to cast it in a new light, and to understand the benefits of your procrastination story—exactly the way it happened.

Every cloud has a silver lining. Every trauma has a gift. Every hardship has at least one lesson that can help make your life better. Let's go back to Alyssa's story. She could end up feeling grateful for what happened by seeing it from this angle.

What I went through with my parents was hard, and I wouldn't wish that on anyone. But it also motivated me to figure out what was going on and why I felt so stuck. Because of what happened, and because of how I eventually handled it, now I feel like I'll become even more successful.

Can you see how Alyssa's acceptance, understanding, and gratitude for what happened will probably lead to higher levels of success in her life?

Here's how I changed my perspective so that now I'm grateful for my procrastination.

I wasted so much time and energy procrastinating during large segments of my life, but I wouldn't change a thing. There's no way I could understand procrastination the way I do now if I hadn't lived as a procrastinator. Now I know procrastination from the inside out, and that allows me to help other procrastinators in ways I never could have without living through it. Ironically, I am extremely thankful I procrastinated because now I can offer different strategies for how people can change. Everything that happened was perfect because it led me to where I am today.

What can you learn from your procrastination story? What lesson does it have to teach you? There may be several lessons you can learn. It's important to identify the silver lining of your procrastination. To look for the gifts of your experiences, the nuggets of wisdom that came out of your delays, no matter how hard it was to live through them.

You may not be able to see all the gifts of your procrastination story—yet. Write them down if you can. At the very least, write down the lessons you have learned so far. Then look for ways to feel grateful for how those lessons can enhance your life. Whenever you feel guilt or regret, or whenever you feel bad about lost time or opportunities, remind yourself of why you're thankful now. Here are some examples.

I'm grateful for my procrastination because I learned that . . .

- waiting until the last minute to get started on my goals is so stressful.
- my avoidance activities don't take me any closer to achieving what I really want.
- my perfectionism keeps me stuck.
- always saying "Yes" to other people means I'm saying "No" to my own goals.
- my procrastination isn't my fault. I'm not lazy or unmotivated. I'm so grateful I can let go of that guilt.

Okay, go back to your paper or get back on your phone or computer and write down the lessons from your procrastination story so far, the ones you're thankful you have learned.

I also suggest that you tell your entire procrastination story to someone else, maybe a close friend or family member, including your happy ending. And tell the last part, your happy ending, to yourself. More than once. Read it out loud. Or stand in front of a mirror, look yourself in the eyes, and say it out loud. Again and again. It may feel awkward or silly, but that's okay. Step outside your comfort zone and try it anyway, at least when you're alone and just by yourself. Visualize what your happy ending will look like. Put pictures on your refrigerator and bathroom mirror that represent your future success.

I used to visualize myself holding a copy of this book, and I would imagine how deeply satisfying that would feel. I would "see" my book listed for sale on Amazon, right along with the cover and description. If you see and feel your happy ending in your mind over and over, and if you repeatedly speak it out loud, it will start to change the pictures you have in your mind about your life as a procrastinator, which will start to pave the way for your happily-ever-after ending to actually come true.

Your Procrastination Story Has a Payoff

As I mentioned before, one of the core principles of psychology is that if you keep doing something again and again, it's because there's a reward or a payoff. You're getting something out of it. If there's no payoff, you will stop doing it. If it doesn't meet a need or a desire, you won't continue.

You can use this principle to change your behavior, just like I did. Earlier in this book I told the story of how I procrastinated on my first job by going to the staff meetings late, then I finally realized that being late made me feel powerful. That feeling of power was a theme in all of my experiences with procrastination. I felt power over other people when I made them wait on me. And I felt powerful just within myself when I waited until the last minute and still managed to pull off mini-miracles by sliding under the wire at the last second. Whether my procrastination involved other people (like arriving late to meetings), or whether it was a situation that only involved me (like waiting to pay my bills), feeling powerful was the payoff.

Thank heavens I already knew that there's nothing wrong with wanting to feel powerful. It's a basic human need that we all have. But it's important to find healthy, constructive ways to feel powerful. Being late or withholding your promises to other people may feel like you're getting the upper hand, but it's disrespectful and can cause major problems in your relationships. It is a form of dominance, not a healthy expression of power.

Empowerment on the other hand, is where we develop our strengths and abilities and express those in constructive ways. When we're empowered, we stand up for our individual rights. When we help others do the same, it becomes mutual empowerment and we all rise together. For example, as a speaker, consultant, and writer, my role is always to help empower others. That is part of why it's so rewarding.

After my staff meeting epiphany, I found healthier and more constructive ways to feel powerful (empowered), both professionally and personally, and that reduced my need to procrastinate by about half. For instance, I became the associate director of the counseling center where I worked, and I got to develop my administrative skills. I wrote policy manuals and brochures, which I enjoyed. I offered new workshops and counseling groups to the students who used our services. In my personal life, I improved my diet, learned new exercise routines, got more into meditation, and completed home improvement projects when I had the time and money.

There are lots of ways to develop new skills, increase your self-confidence, and feel empowered if you look for them. **Ways that take you toward your goals instead of away from them.** Ways that keep you moving toward a more successful future rather than keeping you stuck in your old, dead-end habits.

Later on, I figured out that feeling powerful wasn't the only reward I was getting out of my procrastination. It also provided intensity and challenge. I could lollygag around and spice up even the most routine and boring tasks by adding in emotions like excitement and suspense. If I waited until the last minute to get dressed and out the door, would I make it to class on time? If I went one more day before mailing my electricity bill, would it get there by the due date?

This part of my story falls into the Crisis Maker procrastination style, where I created the crisis and then got to be the hero who always saved the day. My self-created dramas were mostly harmless, except for the ridiculous amounts of stress and wasted energy. Plus, they constantly threw my adrenal glands into overdrive. I sometimes like that feeling of being pumped up, but long-term adrenaline addiction can eventually create health problems because it's a source of chronic internal stress. Some people enjoy thrill-seeking and more dangerous activities that give them the high of an adrenaline overload, like gambling and driving too fast. If you're one of them, just know that it's possible to get your excitement and intensity needs met in safer and more productive ways.

Now I create intensity in my life through carefully chosen personal and professional goals. For example, I experiment with different ways to get better as a speaker and writer, look for more ways to help more people, give more to my personal relationships, find new ways to improve my health, and continue to fine-tune my time management. There's always something else to try, so you can never run out of new challenges. All of these can provide intensity and excitement, depending on how you go about them. If nothing else, put deadlines on your goals and see how quickly and efficiently you can reach them.

After decades of studying procrastination, my own and other people's, after digging into books and journal articles and anything else I could find, I came to the conclusion that no matter what the payoff for your procrastination seems to be on the surface, every act of procrastination includes an underlying attempt to feel powerful. To feel in control, where you're calling the shots. To do things that help you avoid pain or even mild discomfort, and to feel pleasure instead. To feel safe. There's nothing wrong with any of that.

In the final analysis, we all want to be happy. Our procrastination stories tell us at least part of how we are trying to attain that happiness. Are we achieving long-term happiness from a productive, successful life? Or is it fleeting, short-term pleasure from avoidance activities that only give us immediate gratification and a temporary fix?

Procrastination in Relationships

Finding healthy ways to get your basic human needs met also applies to relationships. Couples who are having relationship problems are often caught up in a power struggle without knowing it. For example, one time I spoke on procrastination to a group of men who ranged in age from their sixties into their nineties. I gave my talk, which included my story about how procrastination made me feel powerful. As I watched the faces of the men who were there, I couldn't tell how they were reacting.

After my talk, I asked if anyone had questions. A gentleman raised his hand and said, "Every time we go somewhere, my wife is late. I've tried reminding her of what time we need to leave. I've tried everything I know to do, but nothing works. So now I just go sit in the car and wait for her to come out of the house. Are you telling me that makes her feel powerful?"

The entire room suddenly fell silent. No one moved. I gently but matter-of-factly replied, "If her behavior is a habit, it's because she's getting something out of it. There's a reward or a payoff. Many couples have these kinds of power struggles around procrastination. She may not realize it, but yes, she could be feeling powerful."

In that moment, I could almost see the light bulbs going on in the minds of many of the men in the room. My talk may have increased the power struggle in that one gentleman's marriage. However, my hope is that his new-found awareness was the beginning of his wife's journey to finding healthy ways to feel powerful. Ways that would enhance their relationship instead of creating friction and stress.

If you are in a relationship where there are ongoing conflicts around some type of procrastination, it may be due to an underlying power struggle. Sometimes you will see it in employer-employee relationships, which was the case with me. And like me, your awareness may open the door for positive changes.

You also see this type of struggle all the time in parent-child relationships. The classic example is when parents want their children to clean their rooms, and the children keep resisting and putting it off. Starting around the age of two, children are supposed to start asserting their power and becoming more independent. Both are necessary to develop into well-adjusted adults. It's the responsibility of their parents and other caregivers around them to help children find healthy ways to assert their power by learning skills and becoming competent in areas they can enjoy. Then there's not as much of a need for the power struggles.

When you are the one procrastinating—in your relationships or just in your own personal experiences—and you want a simple and quick technique to stop doing it, ask yourself this question, **"What is the payoff for my procrastination?"** Dig deep inside and be as honest as you can when you answer that question. Then find healthy ways to get that need met. Here's a hint: look for the emotional payoff you're getting. How does your procrastination make you feel? Find productive ways to get that same feeling by moving toward your goals, not away from them. The next chapter includes strategies and techniques to help you do that.

Chapter 3 Highlights

Good for you for reading this far! Your time commitment is commendable. You've hung in there long enough to understand why procrastination isn't your fault. That's a great start. In this chapter, we looked at some of the reasons you procrastinate and why it can be so difficult to overcome. Let's review the main concepts, along with the action steps that were suggested.

1. You are not alone in your struggles to overcome procrastination. At

any given time, "To stop procrastinating" is one of the top reported goals in the *world*.

2. People who understand the reasons they procrastinate are more successful in overcoming it.

3. This book is designed to help you identify the causes of your procrastination and achieve long-term, sustainable behavior change rather than just temporarily fix the symptoms of your repeated delays.

4. Procrastination can be defined as a coping strategy to avoid uncomfortable emotions. The majority of the time, it isn't the task you're avoiding, it's the emotions that go along with it.

5. What you learn before the age of seven—from the people and environment around you—often becomes cemented in your brain as hard-and-fast beliefs, your version of The Truth. These beliefs are often hidden in your subconscious mind, but they can continue to control your thoughts and actions *for the rest of your life* unless you become aware of them and change them.

6. You don't always get what you want. Instead, you usually get what you believe. In other words, your beliefs create your reality.

7. Each of us has a **comfort zone** of what is normal, familiar, and what we are used to. Your subconscious mind wants to keep you safe, which means staying inside your comfort zone. Very often, when you try to move outside this zone, your subconscious mind freaks out and makes you feel afraid that would be too dangerous. So you procrastinate and stay stuck where you've always been.

Action Steps

In the last chapter summary, you were encouraged to take imperfect action in order to complete the recommended activities. Now that you know about your comfort zone and how it works to keep you stuck, throughout the rest of this book, you will also be encouraged to take **uncomfortable action.** Uncomfortable action will help you move into a new normal, to expand your comfort zone so the behavior required to complete your goals starts to become more familiar and less frightening.

1. Review the six procrastination styles: Perfectionist, Dreamer, Worrier, Crisis Maker, Defier, and Pleaser. Can you relate to one or more of these styles? If so, which ones and why?

2. Write down your procrastination story, the one that's embedded in your life story. Next, write a happy ending to your procrastination story and practice saying it out loud. Finally, write down the lessons you have learned from your procrastination story and why you are grateful for them. This activity can be a powerful way to begin moving beyond procrastination.

3. Ask yourself this question, "What is the payoff for my procrastination?" Among other things, be sure to look for the emotional payoff, then find healthy ways to meet that need or desire.

Chapter 4

Outsmart Impulsiveness

Joe Namath was one of the most well-known football quarterbacks in American history. He played for the New York Jets for twelve years and became a household name, recognized almost as much for his partying as for his football prowess. After he retired from football in 1978, Namath's partying continued, and he became an alcoholic. His drinking got so bad that it ruined his marriage and he got lost in his addiction.

Namath realized his life would continue to go downhill if he didn't stop drinking. He figured out there was a certain voice in his head that would tell him to drink. To help him fight that inner voice, Namath decided to name it Slick. By giving it a name and making it more obvious, he could start to say "No" to that voice. It worked, and Namath was finally able to quit. He later said something like, "Slick still whispers every so often, but now that I have a name for him, I listen to him differently."

Giving a name to your inner voices can dramatically increase your awareness of the thoughts that are getting in the way of living your best life. I heard the voice of my procrastination telling me different versions of "You can do it later," but by giving that voice a name, it became easier to stop my dawdling and delays. I knew my procrastination could happen in a millisecond. One second I was sitting at my computer, getting ready to work on an important report. The next second I was scrolling through news sites, caught up in a dopamine rush that instantly blocked any efforts to be productive. My procrastination seemed so quick and so clever that I decided to call that voice Sneaky.

Bringing Sneaky out of the muddle of other thoughts in my head and into more conscious awareness has been one of the keys in helping me reach my goals. The reason it works is because our behavior starts with our thoughts. We need to change our thoughts before we can change our behavior and *do* something different. I suggest that you give your inner voice of procrastination a name. It can be a fun way to start breaking your bad habits, so think of some possibilities. Just make sure the names you consider aren't too negative, but more descriptive and even playful.

The Importance of Mindset

Up until now in this book, we have mostly been focusing on your mindset, the beliefs that determine your thoughts, emotions and attitudes about yourself and your procrastination. Because our beliefs also determine our behavior, mindset is often the best place to start when you want to change and start doing something different.

In her book *Mindset: The New Psychology of Success*, psychologist Carol Dweck describes new psychological breakthroughs with the identification of two types of mindset. People who have a **fixed mindset** believe their potential is limited, that potential is established at birth and can't be increased or improved. No amount of learning or effort or hard work will help them become more intelligent, more talented, more athletic, or more capable, so they don't try to get better. These people are often hesitant to try new things, because if they don't succeed right away, they think it's because they are incapable of ever being successful, which makes them feel inadequate. Other people have more of what's called a **growth mindset**. These people believe their potential is unlimited. They thrive on challenges and love to learn how to increase their abilities and improve in all areas of their lives. Whether or not you believe that lifelong learning and improvement are possible will become your self-fulfilling prophecy. In other words, **what you believe shapes what you achieve**.

Most of us have what I call a **mixed mindset**. We believe that through learning and effort, we can improve in some but probably not all parts of our lives. There are still some areas where we have glass ceilings that stay out of reach. For example, maybe you can't seem to stay happy for very long. Or you can't increase your income past a certain amount. Maybe you always gain back the weight you lost. Many times these ceilings remain invisible until you try to break through them. Nonetheless, they still keep you trapped somewhere below your potential.

Because you are reading this book, I assume that you have a growth mindset when it comes to overcoming your procrastination. You believe you can change your unproductive habits and learn how to stop your unnecessary delays. Having a growth mindset when it comes to your procrastination will help you apply the techniques in this book. It will also help you get through the inevitable challenges along the road to your success in all the other areas of your life.

Highly successful people usually have a growth mindset which is based on several core empowering beliefs. I've seen different versions of these beliefs with employees, entrepreneurs, students, athletes, and artists. These may not be conscious beliefs, but they at least open the door to improve your life. In general, successful people believe

The future can be better than the present. I have the power to make it better.

Right now, ask yourself if you believe those two statements are true for you. Do you believe your future can be better, and you can make that happen? If you hesitate before answering, there will be lots of opportunities to develop a more solid and unwavering growth mindset in the coming chapters. That's because according to Dweck's research, **we can choose which mindset we want to believe**. When you choose a growth mindset over a fixed mindset, you can start to succeed more often. You start believing in yourself and your own abilities to make things happen. And your beliefs largely determine the outcome of your efforts. Learning and succeeding become fun again, just like when you were a child.

If you are a chronic procrastinator, it almost goes without saying that you have disempowering, limiting beliefs. Maybe you are aware of your limiting beliefs, and maybe you're not, but it's almost guaranteed that they are a major root cause of your procrastination. In the next chapter, we will cover the quickest and most recently discovered strategies to transform your limiting beliefs into empowering ones. But first, I want to help you understand another part of your subconscious mind—in addition to limiting beliefs—that can keep you procrastinating. In this chapter, I will show you how to bypass this part of your mind through simple brain hacks that can give you immediate success with your goals. This step is important, because even if you have empowering beliefs, what we cover in this chapter can still cause you to procrastinate.

The following techniques will be extremely valuable after you transform you limiting beliefs. But I am teaching them to you now because the quick success they bring can boost your self-confidence and give you extra motivation and incentive to keep going. They also allow you to start tapping into dopamine so you can start feeling good about your progress. Right now. These techniques can help you add hours of productive time to each and every day, so let's dive in.

How Impulsiveness Contributes to Your Procrastination

When I first started studying procrastination in the 1980s, therapists believed that people procrastinated because of fear of failure. They didn't want to try because they didn't want to fail. But through working with their clients, therapists found that some people procrastinated out of a fear of success, which is another version of fear of failure but with a little different twist. These procrastinators are afraid that success will bring unwanted consequences. Maybe other people will be jealous. Or maybe people will only like them because they are rich or successful in other ways. People might place expectations on them to keep succeeding or do even better, and what if they can't meet those expectations? There would only be one place to go from a pinnacle of success, and that is a fall from grace.

But then Piers Steel came along and turned those theories upside down. Steel was a faculty member in the psychology department at the University of Calgary in Canada. He developed a way to analyze all the procrastination studies that were available at the time, over 800 of them, and to factor out the causes of procrastination that were found in each one. What he discovered was beyond surprising. The main reason people in these studies procrastinated was because of **impulsiveness.** What? Impulsiveness? If that's true, then what makes us so impulsive? If we can find the answer to that question, if we can determine the underlying cause of impulsiveness, then maybe we can short-circuit that factor and find easier ways to stop putting things off.

As procrastinators, we are very fortunate to be living in this day and age, because there has been an explosion of brain research in the past twenty years. Researchers have learned more in that time about how our brains work than in the past 100 years combined. They have discovered the part of the brain that is responsible for impulsiveness and the part of the brain that's in charge of controlling it. That means we can look for ways to work *with* our brains so they help us achieve our goals rather than continuing to sabotage our efforts.

As you might imagine, how impulsive you are is largely determined by your beliefs. But impulsiveness can also simply become a bad habit, something you do without thinking. For instance, you may believe you are a strong person, capable of controlling your impulses most of the time. You may find it hard to believe you're the kind of person who would put off doing important things and instead impulsively scroll through your phone—for hours. Day after day. And yet that may be what you do. You probably feel bad about it, but you may still do it. It's so easy to slide into that rut and stay there.

When you do things that contradict what you believe about yourself, you often pay a price with guilt. The emotional toll it takes is expensive. Not only do you feel bad about your procrastination, but guilt is one of those emotions that can drain your physical, mental, and emotional energy and make it harder to get other things done.

The suggestions in this chapter will help you tap into your empowering beliefs, let go of your guilt, and strengthen your growth mindset. Through techniques like giving your procrastination a name, these suggestions will also describe lots of ways to start breaking any bad habits you might have where impulsiveness makes your procrastination worse, in spite of your empowering beliefs.

We're Hardwired to Be Impulsive

What makes you automatically check your phone much more than you need to throughout the day? What makes you grab the TV remote so quickly and opt for television time instead of doing what you planned to do? Why do you reach for that candy bar at the checkout counter even though you are trying to lose ten pounds?

We already know that the subconscious mind is responsible for our beliefs. But keeping us safe by using our beliefs is only part of its job. It also tries to keep us safe from any kind of impending physical danger, any threat to our physical safety that would require us to either fight or run away. The subconscious mind contains an automatic safety switch that doesn't require us to think—just act. It purposely bypasses our thinking in the threat of the moment to ensure that we make it through the immediate danger. In other words, at times, it acts completely on impulse.

The part of the subconscious mind that contains these impulsive survival instincts is called the **limbic system**. Located in the central section of the brain, it is the part that contains our basic drive to avoid pain (and danger) and to seek pleasure. This network of structures includes the

amygdala and several other parts of the brain which share responsibility for emotions, memories, and motivation. The amygdala itself is a small almond-shaped structure located deep within the brain, and it contains some our most primal instincts for self-preservation, including our fight, flight, or freeze instincts. These instincts play an important role in how we handle fear and form new habits. Also contained in the limbic system is a small but mighty component called the **nucleus accumbens**, which is the actual source of dopamine and provides the feel-good emotions that happen when dopamine is released. Without this entire system, we wouldn't be able to stay motivated and experience the pleasure that comes from learning and making progress on our goals.

It's interesting that the limbic system is also responsible for the hunger drive, especially given the fact that so many people impulsively overeat. But that makes sense, because this system runs on immediate gratification. It only knows present time (not past or future), and it wants what it wants when it wants it, which is always now. Spontaneous, creative, and delightful (at times), it thrives on what is pleasurable, easy, and fun in the moment. Because of these qualities, I think of the limbic system as our **Inner Child** and more affectionately, the **Fun One**.

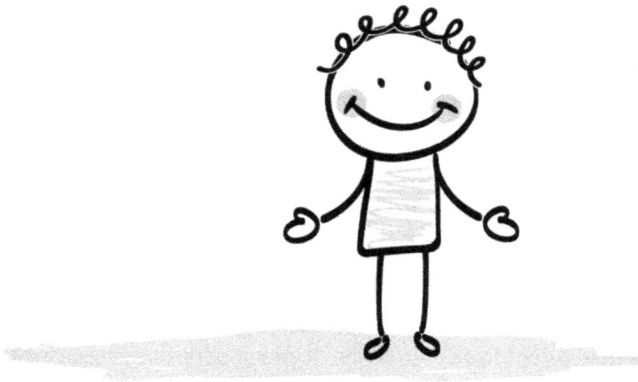

INNER CHILD, the FUN ONE

Just like with all children, our Inner Child can be an absolute joy to be around, but only if it has rules to follow and is kept within certain boundaries. Otherwise, it can turn into an unruly spoiled brat. By nature, the Inner Child wants to eat all the candy in the candy store. Right now.

If a little is good, a lot is better. It wants to do enjoyable things and keep doing them way past any reasonable period of time. Once it discovers the high that comes from a dopamine rush, it may keep going with no regard for any other activities that need to get done. When it is in the moment of this pleasurable high, it's as if all the other things on your to-do list don't even exist.

Without structure and healthy guidelines, the Fun One can go too far with its indulgences, and that's when it turns into what I call the **Party Child**. All of us have a Party Child inside of us that needs an adult around to keep it from overindulging and getting carried away. Some people don't feel comfortable with Inner Child references or activities. If that's the case for you, you can think of your Inner Child as the impulsive part of your brain or your subconscious mind.

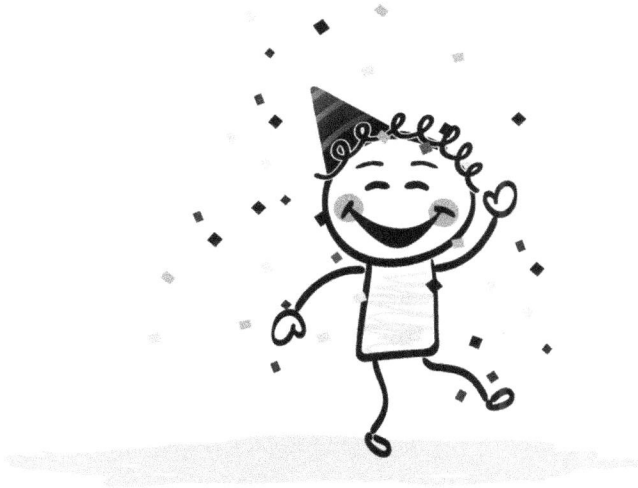

INNER CHILD, the PARTY CHILD

Your conscious awareness is the adult we all need. Called the **prefrontal cortex**, this conscious thinking part of the mind is located at the front of the brain (just behind the forehead). It contains our willpower and controls our impulsive reactions. Sometimes referred to as the executive function part of our brain, it's in charge of self-control, decision-making, and problem-solving. It helps us look back into the past and learn from our mistakes, and it can anticipate future consequences of our actions. That means that the prefrontal cortex helps us plan strategies for success then control our behavior for long enough to reach our goals. Rational and responsible, I call this part of the brain our **Inner Adult**. And because our

Inner Adult contains the abilities we need to make our dreams come true, I fondly refer to it as the **Dream Maker**.

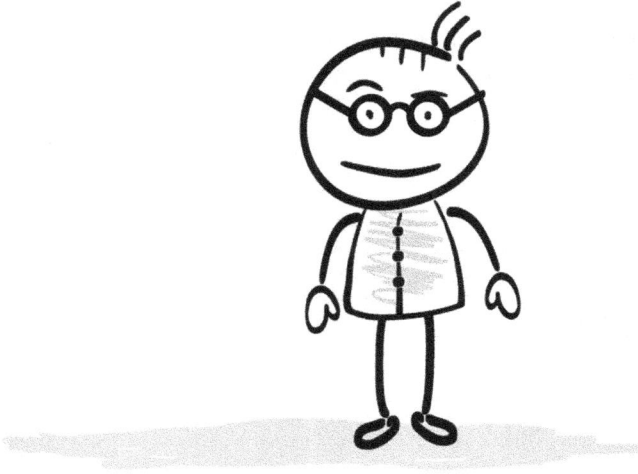

INNER ADULT, the DREAM MAKER

The prefrontal cortex doesn't fully develop until we're around the age of twenty-five. People younger than that aren't able to foresee future consequences and will tend to believe they are invincible. When you hear about teenagers and young adults who do stupid things that get them hurt or killed, have compassion for them instead of being judgmental. Their undeveloped minds probably couldn't let them see what might happen. That's not to say they shouldn't be held accountable for their actions. But the bad choices, impulsivity, and general lack of patience of young people need to be seen in a different developmental context than those of adults.

Once the prefrontal cortex is fully developed, then just like our Inner Child, our Inner Adult can get carried away and go too far. It may want to focus and concentrate for too long, without breaks, and without providing the Inner Child with any play time. I call this part the **Harsh Taskmaster**, and it has the potential to ruin almost anything.

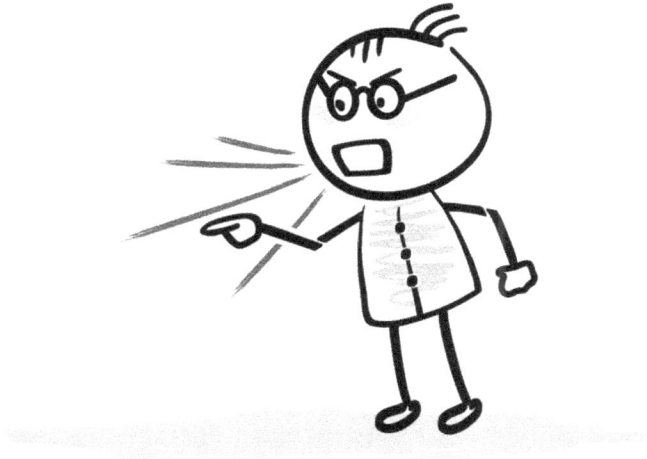

INNER ADULT, the HARSH TASKMASTER

Your Inner Adult needs to stay within healthy boundaries as well. You can't just push and push and push and not expect there to be some kind of backlash. If you work too long and too hard all day long, don't be surprised if you sit down in front of the television when you get home and mindlessly eat an entire bag of chips. When that happens, it's probably just your Inner Child looking for some pleasure. Your prefrontal cortex takes a much-needed break, you stop consciously thinking about what you're doing, and your impulsive, feel-good limbic system takes over. An easy way to remember this is that **the limbic system is the emotional part of your brain and the prefrontal cortex is your reasoning.**

In this example, the Inner Child took over after the work was done. When we procrastinate, the Inner Child usually interferes with our work before we get started. You will impulsively check your email when you need to work on that report. You will wander into the kitchen to look for something to eat when it's time to work on your taxes. You will decide to post to Instagram when you had planned to send off that email.

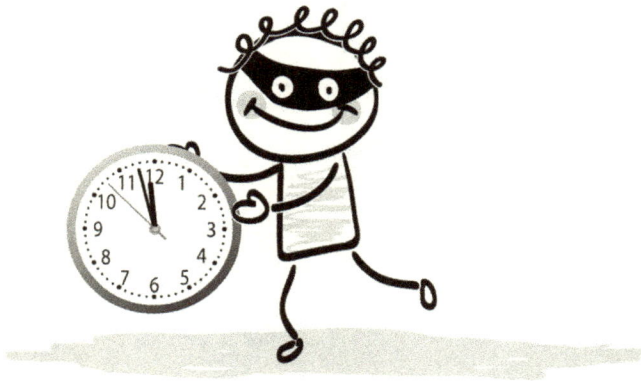

These conflicts may be more likely to happen if your Harsh Taskmaster is too driven and regularly gets carried away. The Inner Child knows that you will probably work too long and too hard, so it is likely to rebel and steal your time by doing one of your avoidance activities. Even if your Harsh Taskmaster has learned to set reasonable time limits on work, your Inner Child may impulsively jump into an avoidance activity, especially if what you want to do is unpleasant—possibly boring, frustrating, or overwhelming. Our rational and responsible Inner Adult is willing to forego temporary pleasure for long-term gain, but our Inner Child just wants enjoyable play time, now. In other words, our prefrontal cortex and our limbic system often compete and frequently become head-to-head opponents in the Inner Game.

How can we resolve these conflicts? What can we do to keep our impulsive Inner Child from stealing our time again and again? Some people will try to shame their Inner Child into obedience and submission. They will say mean and hateful things to themselves like, "You idiot! I can't believe you just wasted all that time. What's wrong with you?" You wouldn't admonish a young child the way you mentally beat up on yourself, but this is sometimes how we talk to ourselves. As we discussed earlier however, guilt and shame only make things worse. They intensify the battle between the Inner Child and the Inner Adult. The Inner Child will often dig its heels in even deeper, and you will probably either stay at your current level of stuckness or become even more entrenched in that battle.

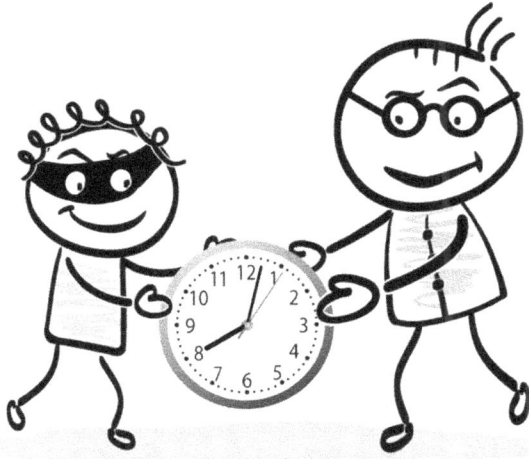

It is crucial to understand that most of the time, the Inner Child not only wants to play, but also just wants to feel safe. It's not a bad kid. Sometimes it can just be scared. Or it feels lost because it doesn't have any guidelines. Yes, it wants to feel good all the time, but eating too much candy doesn't make you feel good in the long run, and the Inner Child needs a strong and loving Inner Adult to set healthy boundaries and make it feel safe.

Children thrive when they have boundaries and clear expectations. When children act out and misbehave, they are often begging their parents to set limits on their behavior, because reasonable rules make them feel secure. They want to know how to please their parents so they will get their love, attention, and approval. The same guidelines apply to your Inner Child. If you can provide healthy boundaries and communicate with your Inner Child with love and acceptance, your child will learn it is safe, it will know what's expected, and will be more likely to cooperate with your Inner Adult.

In the absence of these healthy boundaries, many people live as if there's a five-year-old tyrant with an ironclad grip on the steering wheel of their lives, driving them around from one impulsive indulgence to another. They continually procrastinate, overeat, drink too much, abuse prescription medications, gamble, shop, or play video games. They never realize that as an adult, they can use their conscious awareness to take back their power by setting reasonable limits for their Inner Child. Perhaps they realize they have that choice, but they don't know how to set healthy boundaries or diffuse that inner power struggle. The rest of this book includes all kinds of suggestions for how to create healthy limits for dealing with your procrastination. Many of these strategies can also be helpful with addictions and other impulsive overindulgences as well. These recommendations are based on the underlying principle that

The goal is to create win-win situations between your Inner Child and your Inner Adult.

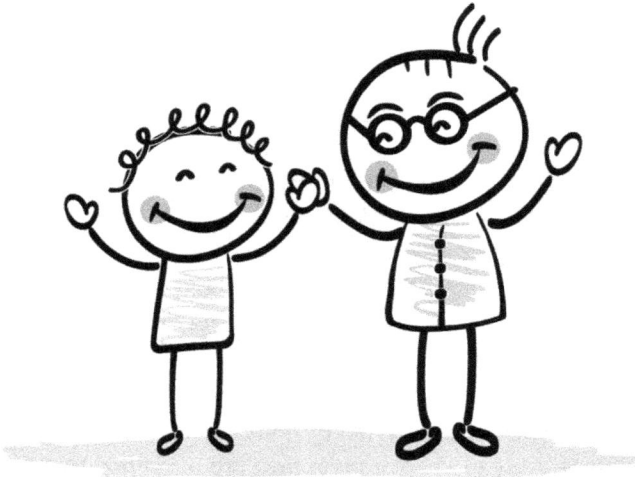

Most long-term goals that are worth doing—goals that have the ability to change your future for the better—require repeated periods of focus and concentration. In order to spend that much time focusing on those kinds of goals, we need both our Inner Adult with its clarity and willpower, and our Inner Child, which connects us to our playfulness, creativity, positive emotions, and dopamine. Without an adequate supply of dopamine from the Inner Child, we won't have the motivation to keep going. Besides, we can't disconnect from our limbic system at will. And we wouldn't want to. The dopamine and emotions it provides are what make our learning and progress enjoyable. The limbic system helps lead us into a future where success breeds success. Overall, we need to create a healthy **balance** between these two parts of our brains.

Right now, let's look at some simple and practical ways to control your impulsive Inner Child while at the same time giving it healthy play time. These activities will help you create more balance in your brain by leveling the playing field and giving your Inner Adult better odds of winning. They will also provide some immediate success with your goals, which will give you more incentive to keep going.

Use This Quick-Fix Technique for Immediate Results

What we now know from brain science is that your prefrontal cortex contains your willpower, and your willpower functions like a muscle. It is strongest when you first start to use it, but it gets weaker the longer you use it at any given time. Think about lifting weights. When you first start, it probably feels easy. But as you keep lifting, your muscles begin to get tired, and it becomes harder to keep going. There is a limit to how much weightlifting you can do all at once. The same is true for willpower. It is a limited resource that is not sustainable over a long period of time on any given day.

However, it's also true that willpower gets stronger if you keep using it day after day. Athletes can only work their muscles so much over one day's time. But if they keep exercising a little each day over several weeks, their muscles eventually get stronger. The same thing happens with willpower. If you practice strengthening your willpower each day, then over time, it will eventually get stronger. The key is to repeatedly give it a good workout.

First thing in the morning, your willpower is at its strongest and better able to handle the myriad of distractions and temptations that might get you off track from what you planned. You drive right past the coffee shop on your way to work. You politely say "No thanks" to the office goodies that are loaded with calories. You ignore your itching desire to hop on Facebook and see what your friends are up to. But as the day goes on and you have to keep using your willpower to stay focused on your goals, it starts getting weaker. By the end of the day, the strength of your willpower is at its lowest point. You had to make thousands of decisions and resist hundreds of impulsive urges since waking up that morning. The evening and nighttime hours are when you will be most likely to eat that bowl of ice cream that you swore you weren't going to eat. Or binge on late night television shows when you need to go to sleep. If you practice resisting temptations however, over time your willpower will get stronger, even at the end of the day.

This means that it will be easier to use your willpower to focus and concentrate at the beginning of your day. I call this invaluable, prized period of the day the **golden hours**, because if you use those first few hours to work on your most important goals, you can get more done in less time. Your prefrontal cortex will help you out with not only more willpower, but with better clarity, decision-making, and problem-solving. Besides that, most people have more control over what they do at the start of their day than later on when all kinds of unexpected things can impose on their time.

You may be thinking *But I'm not a morning person*. And that is a valid point. Each of us has a natural **internal prime time**, the time in the day when we have the most energy and find it easiest to concentrate and be productive. I used to ask my university students, "When is your prime time?" Out of thousands of students, the majority said they were morning people. Only a relatively few said they were mid-day people, and the rest said they worked best at night.

Over the many years I asked about prime time, I noticed that the number of students who said they were morning people seemed to decline. When I questioned the students about their sleep patterns, they often told me they were staying up late to catch up on social media. It became almost impossible for them to get up early when they regularly went to sleep so late. I've also worked with clients who slept enough hours at night, but they were consuming too much caffeine during the day or drinking alcohol too close to bedtime, which compromised the quality of their sleep. They didn't feel rested in the morning and found it hard to focus on anything other than their habitual morning routines. Using the golden hours was not an option.

All of us have natural circadian rhythms that influence our internal prime time. However, you can learn how to take advantage of the golden hours—even if you aren't naturally a morning person—by changing your nightly sleep habits. More people could be productive in the morning if they went to bed earlier and got get plenty of quality sleep. You can see this happening in reverse: more people become night owls when they go to bed late, wake up late, and don't feel rested.

No matter when you naturally tend to have your prime time, that doesn't change the fact that your willpower is strongest at the beginning of the day. The good news is that you can train your mind to work on your most important goals first thing in the morning, even if it doesn't come naturally at first. It may take some time, but with repetition you can start to use those golden hours to become more successful with whatever goals are important to you. If you are currently a night owl and your most productive time is at the end of the day, using the golden hours may feel like a big stretch for you right now. That's okay. However, by making small changes, you may eventually learn how to take advantage of this golden time, so stay open to possibilities.

You can start with this experiment. When you first get up in the morning, see if you can work on your most important priority. Maybe you can start by working for ten minutes during the golden hours. If that's too hard, you can count even five minutes of focused time as a success. The objective is to start training yourself to use the golden hours to make progress on something important. If you make a good faith effort to use the golden hours first thing in the morning and can't seem to make it work, I encourage you to identify when you are naturally more focused and productive. Then find ways to use that time to work on your top priorities and most important goals, scheduling your other activities around it to preserve that time when you can.

Many people check their phones the second they wake up. If you use your phone as your alarm clock, you're already looking at your phone and probably already holding your phone first thing in the morning. You may be in the habit of quickly scrolling through texts, emails, social media, or the news, which means you start your day online. "Just a few minutes" to see what's been posted overnight can easily become 10 minutes or more. **This is the worst thing you can do.** The instant you go online, you get a big dopamine rush, and your mind immediately craves more. Your limbic system takes over, and your impulsive Inner Child is now driving the car. Your Party Child just won the first round of the Inner Game for that day. And you probably haven't even gotten out of bed.

Not only that, but once you go online, your prefrontal cortex will take a back seat, it will get flooded with dopamine, and **that will make it harder to focus and concentrate—for the whole rest of the day!** Now you have to use your willpower to not only steer yourself through the normal distractions and resistance to working on your goals, but you have to overcome the craving for more dopamine. By going online, you just stacked the odds in favor of your Party Child, making it more likely you will struggle to overcome your procrastination until the next morning. That's because sleep gives your brain a chance to recover from too much dopamine during the day. Sleep diminishes your dopamine craving and gives you a fresh start. But all of this can be avoided if you don't go onto the internet until *after* you have worked on your goal during the golden hours, even if it's for a short amount of time.

Start Your Day in a Proactive Position

As if creating a massive dopamine craving weren't bad enough, going online also puts you in a **reactive position**, reacting to other people's messages. It makes you start thinking about what other people have posted instead of thinking about your own plans and goals. It takes you away from your goals, not toward them. What matters most here is for you to start the day in a **proactive position,** taking charge of your time by focusing on you and your priorities. This will set the tone for the entire rest of your day.

If you decide to work on a personal goal first thing in the morning, it may mean getting up earlier. That's fine, as long as you also go to bed earlier and don't cut back on your sleep. One of my all-time favorite books on time management was written by Alan Lakein. With a family and a busy career to juggle, Lakein decided that early morning hours would provide his best writing time. He was already in the habit of getting up at 5:00 and working until 7:00 every morning, so he used that time to write most of his book. It was definitely worth it. *How to Get Control of Your Time and Your Life* went on to sell millions of copies and became a classic in the field.

If your important goal is related to your job, going into the office early when nobody else is around can help you avoid interruptions and take advantage of the golden hours. You may also be able to start working at your regular time and just carve out some morning hours to work on your top priority. For example, Claire, a mid-level manager, used this strategy to gain an additional three hours of work time during her day. She immediately understood how a big rush of dopamine first thing in the morning made it harder to concentrate from then on, so she decided to try a new schedule. Claire stayed off the internet before going into her office. Then instead of checking her email when she first got to work and throughout the day as she normally did, she waited and checked her email at noon each day. Without the constant interruptions and dopamine hits of going online throughout the morning, she was able to zero in on her work projects, and her productivity soared.

I want you to be successful with productively using your golden hours because this is one of the quickest and easiest ways to make progress on your goals. It is a simple brain hack that can help you maximize the use of your willpower and minimize your impulsive urges. You can slip through the back door and get started on your goals without a direct confrontation with your tendencies to resist. You can tiptoe past your sleeping Inner Child to keep from waking it up and setting off a crying spell that delays or derails your plans for the rest of the day.

If You're Still Stuck, Try These Techniques

Once you get a little experience in using the golden hours, it will give you undeniable, living proof that you can be successful. Your self-worth will increase, and you will have more self-confidence going into all of your future goals. However, if you find it difficult to spend even five minutes working on your goal before you check your phone or go online, that means it is time to do some problem solving and figure out how to keep procrastination from taking away the best time of the day to do what's important to you.

When you get stuck and find it hard to stop procrastinating on your goals, the fastest route to success is usually to first try making changes to your Outer Game. Experiment with different changes in your environment that will make it easier for you to succeed. The goal here is to **make it easy to do the right thing and hard to do the wrong thing**. You can switch things around in your physical world or rearrange your schedule to change *when* you do certain tasks.

More often than not, overcoming procrastination is a matter of timing. It involves changing the time of day you use to achieve your goal. Your Inner Child and your Inner Adult still get to do what they each want to do, but play time comes later in the day, after your Inner Adult has had a chance to productively focus and concentrate. Here are some suggestions for maximizing your use of the golden hours.

- **Avoid your phone.**
  If you are using your cell phone to wake up in the morning, start using an alarm clock instead.
- **Silence your phone.**
  Turn your phone off the night before or put it on airplane or silent mode so you're not distracted by notifications.
- **Hide your phone.**
  Keep your phone out of sight until you have finished your five minutes (or more). Maybe keep it in a drawer overnight, or at least put something over it so you can't see it. Just the sight of your phone

will probably be a temptation to automatically check it. Some people find that they need to put their phone in a room they don't normally go into in the morning to avoid the urge to pick it up.

If you're worried about missing an emergency call, use the Do Not Disturb settings on your phone to allow calls from certain contacts. Most Do Not Disturb functions will also override your block if you get two calls from the same person within three minutes, so you can let your emergency contacts know this in advance.

- **Block tempting sites.**
  If your downfall is opening your favorite online sites either on your phone or computer, find an app that will either block your most tempting sites or make them harder to open because you must go through several steps.

At times, just making a few simple Outer Game changes will be enough for you to be successful with your goal. If that's not enough, then experiment with Inner Game techniques until you find what works. Here are some internal, mental changes to try.

- **Make a promise in advance.**
  If your goal involves working on your computer, find a way to avoid clicking on the online temptations that would release dopamine. For example, promise yourself in advance that you will only open those sites *after* you have completed your five minutes.

- **Use self-talk to your advantage.**
  You can coach yourself with your internal dialog, through what you say to yourself. Make up some positive self-talk to use when you first get up in the morning. You may even want to write out a few key sentences to help guide you through those first five minutes. Things like, "Be strong right now and focus for five minutes. That's all you need to do." Or, "Stay focused and just open the file you need to work on." Either out loud or silently to yourself, repeat your key sentence(s) like a mantra until you get started on your goal.

- **Say "Not now."**
  If you find yourself opening any other programs than the one you had planned to work on, simply correct your Inner Child by saying, "Not now. Just give me five minutes to focus on my goal, then you can go online."

I've found that saying "**Not now**" followed by a promise of when my Inner Child can do whatever she wants makes it easier for her to wait. A simple "No" told to a child can often be heard as "Not ever" and can trigger rebellion. So I promise my Inner Child a specific time when she can do what she wants. And I keep my promise. The last thing I want to do is start breaking my Inner Adult promises, because then my Inner Child won't believe me when I promise her play time, and she will be more likely to resist me later on.

- **Speak to your procrastination by saying its name.**
What name can you think of that would describe your procrastination? Again, please don't give that inner voice a name that is too judgmental or harsh, but something lighter or even funny. Remember, you need that part of yourself—which is usually your impulsive Inner Child— to give your life creative energy and emotional spark. It's what makes your life fun.

If you start to procrastinate, speak to your procrastination by the name you gave it, either through a dialog in your head or through actual spoken words. I will often start talking out loud, firmly but with an element of playfulness, by saying something like, "Sneaky, I see you. Not now. You can play later, after I finish working on my goal." This kind of dialog makes your procrastination more obvious and brings it out of your impulsive limbic system and into the conscious awareness of your prefrontal cortex. That will give your Inner Adult better odds of winning that particular round of the Inner Game.

- **Start where you are.**
If you find it difficult to focus on your goal for more than just a few minutes, then that is your starting point. Let's say your goal is to exercise more. If you can only ignore your phone for a few minutes, maybe you can do ten jumping jacks. Do whatever you can, but you may be surprised to find that once you start, it's easier than you thought to keep going. You might be able to exercise for eight minutes when your goal was only two minutes. Maybe the next day you can work out for twelve minutes when you only planned to exercise for five.

As you have probably discovered, **the first few minutes of working on any goal are usually the hardest**. That is when your focus has been on something else and your internal resistance is the strongest. Knowing this in advance can help you plan several Outer Game and Inner Game strategies to help you get past those first few minutes. Once you get going, your Inner Adult is in the driver's seat and your prefrontal cortex starts getting dopamine from making progress on your goal. At first, it probably won't be as big of a dopamine hit as mindlessly scrolling the internet and focusing on someone else's news, but you will be in a proactive position, moving toward your goal instead of away from it.

If you can't resist looking at your phone for even two minutes, then consider this quote from author Jen Sincero,

In order to kick ass you must first lift up your foot.

You will need to exert some effort to change your bad habits. The best way I've found to do that is to prepare in advance for how to be successful. Think through the situations that you know will be hard for you and find ways to switch up the factors in the Outer Game and the Inner Game so they stack up in your favor. To help you get started, here's one more suggestion.

- **Give your Inner Child healthy play time every day.**
  What does your Inner Child enjoy doing? What feeds your body and mind, helps you relax, and leaves you in a good mood? Is it physical exercise like bike riding, working out, or walking? Maybe you enjoy spending time on social media or watching television or a movie. Maybe it's a hobby, watching or playing sports, gardening, reading, enjoying music, or playing video games. Maybe meditation soothes your soul. Or spending time with family. Or going to a restaurant or simply talking with friends. Or playing with children or pets. Be careful about play time that involves eating or spending money, because those can lead to unhealthy and expensive indulgences.

If at all possible, build healthy play time into every day. This will make your Inner Child a much happier little kid to start with. Plus, you can use those same activities as rewards for good behavior. If you promise enjoyable play time in the near future, your Inner Child is more likely to be patient as you work on your Inner Adult goals. With a few exceptions, plan to have play time *after* you have taken advantage of the golden hours. But if for example, your Inner Child enjoys working out, and your top priority goal is to exercise more, it may be best to work out first thing in the morning. In general, though, save your play time for later in the day.

Eliminate the Cause Instead of Treating the Symptoms

We all know the symptoms of procrastination. The clever maneuvers that waste our time, take us away from our goals, and rob us of untold opportunities to enjoy a better life. We're all too familiar with the procrastination activities that don't resolve the internal power struggle, but instead allow the battle in our minds to continue. Chronic procrastinators know that using Outer Game techniques like time management and goal setting usually don't work to "treat" these symptoms. They don't make the symptoms go away. Outer Game techniques usually only work for chronic procrastinators when they also address the underlying cause of procrastination, when they take into account the parts of the brain that contribute to procrastination in the first place.

In this chapter, we have explored several parts of the brain that contribute to our endless delays. Primarily the limbic system, but also the prefrontal cortex when our Inner Adult gets carried away and turns into the Harsh Taskmaster. But here's the deal. Your limiting beliefs set the stage for you to fall victim to your impulsive urges and your overly driven Inner Adult. By the same token, strong empowering beliefs can help you override your impulsive urges. For now, just imagine what it would be like if you had rock-solid, empowering, underlying core beliefs like

*I am infinitely resourceful
in reaching my goals.
I keep my eye on the prize
and just keep going.*

Or this one,

My success is inevitable.

Remember, in general our beliefs create our reality. We almost never get what we want unless we have an underlying belief that supports our success. The next chapter provides tools, techniques, and strategies to help you develop the kinds of beliefs that will give you unshakable self-confidence and unstoppable momentum. I'm so excited for you to keep learning how to take back your power and become the shining superstar you are meant to be.

Also, good job for reading this far. You're doing great!

Chapter 4 Highlights

This chapter describes how your brain is hardwired to be impulsive, and how impulsiveness often causes you to procrastinate. It also provides lots of techniques to bypass the impulsive parts of your brain and start doing what you want to do. Here are some of the main points.

1. Highly successful people usually have a strong **growth mindset** and believe that through their own efforts, they have the power to make their future better. In contrast, people who have a **fixed mindset** believe that no amount of effort on their part will help them become more capable of improving their future.

2. According to over 800 research studies, the main factor that contributes to our procrastination is **impulsiveness**. Empowering beliefs can help prevent impulsiveness, but impulsiveness can cause you to procrastinate despite empowering beliefs.

3. Scientists have discovered the part of the brain that is responsible for impulsiveness is the limbic system, and the part of the brain that's in charge of controlling it is the prefrontal cortex. That means you can look for ways to work *with* your brain so it helps you achieve your goals rather than sabotaging your efforts.

4. I call our impulsive limbic system the **Inner Child** and our responsible prefrontal cortex the **Inner Adult**. These two parts of the brain are usually in conflict when we procrastinate. Our impulsive Inner Child wants immediate gratification and to feel good—all the time. Our responsible Inner Adult can provide boundaries for the Inner Child and help us achieve our long-term goals.

5. We need both our Inner Child and our Inner Adult to live successful lives, so it is important to create a healthy and balanced relationship between the two. That's why you will find that many successful people work hard and play hard.

6. Our willpower is contained in the prefrontal cortex. Willpower functions like a muscle. The longer you use it in any one session on any given day, the weaker the muscle will be at the end of that session or day. However, if you practice strengthening your willpower

muscle a little each day—day after day for several weeks—it will get stronger. Also remember that your willpower is strongest in the morning and weakest at night.

7. You can use both Outer Game and Inner Game techniques to work on your top priorities during the morning hours when your willpower, focus, and concentration are the strongest. I call this morning time the **golden hours**.

Action Steps

The action steps recommended in this chapter are designed to help you move past your impulsiveness so your life isn't run by your Inner Child. For example, these steps will help eliminate some of the temptations to use your cell phone as an avoidance activity. They will also help you create a healthy relationship between your Inner Child and your Inner Adult. As before, the goal is for you to take imperfect action (don't get caught up in perfectionism) and to take uncomfortable action. Experiment with the following, even if some of these steps feel uncomfortable or awkward.

1. Give your procrastination a name. Nothing too negative, but more descriptive and playful. Then talk to it. Out loud. Be kind and respectful but firm when you need to be.

2. Do not use your phone as an alarm clock. Do not check your phone until you've taken advantage of the golden hours to focus on your top priorities.

3. Stay off the internet first thing in the morning. As soon as you go online each morning, you get a shot of dopamine and create a craving for more. This makes it harder to focus and concentrate for the whole rest of the day.

4. Save play for later in the day, after your Inner Adult has had a chance to productively focus and concentrate. Overcoming procrastination is often a matter of timing. It involves changing the time of day you use to achieve your goals. Your Inner Child and your Inner Adult still get to do what they each want to do, but play time comes later in the day. Find the techniques in this chapter that help you do that.

Chapter 5

Strategies to Stop Procrastinating

Victor Hugo, the French author of many famous novels, including *Les Misérables*, was a notorious procrastinator. One time he had a deadline to complete a book, but he didn't feel like writing. In order to stop himself from leaving his house, he decided to lock away his clothes and only wear a shawl until the book was done. It worked, and he completed *The Hunchback of Notre Dame* ahead of time.

Other well-known procrastinators include the remarkable architect Frank Loyd Wright, the gifted painter Leonardo da Vinci—even the Dalai Lama during his younger years. And the story goes that the musical virtuoso, Wolfgang Amadeus Mozart, wrote the overture for his famous opera *Don Giovanni* the night before its debut, leaving no time for even a single rehearsal.

Fortunately, none of us has to wait as long or take such drastic measures as some of the procrastinators who have come before us. With the more recent information that has been discovered through neuroscience, coaching, and psychology, we can now find ways to work *with* our brains to overcome our unnecessary delays. But these previous procrastinators have taught us an important lesson. Clearly, overcoming procrastination is not a matter of intelligence. Even geniuses have had their share of struggles.

If it's not IQ though, then what allows us to finally break free? What strategies will give us advantages to win the Inner Game so we don't have to continue to struggle or resort to extreme Outer Game maneuvers? This chapter provides more answers to that question.

Use Your Detective Mindset

Procrastination is often called a **time thief** because it steals our time. But that's not all it steals. It robs us of our goals and dreams, the very things we want for ourselves now and in the future. It can hijack our health and cheat us out of living this life in a body that allows us to enjoy our goals and dreams when we are able to reach them. It can block us from achieving the **outer wealth** of more money and the material possessions, the choices, and the freedom that money can buy. It can also steal our **inner wealth**, the peace, happiness ,and fulfillment that come from a life well lived. The research on procrastination is clear: non-procrastinators are happier, healthier, and wealthier. Yes, the stakes for overcoming your procrastination are high.

The strategies I describe in the rest of this chapter can help you stop your needless delays. But the strategies won't work without some degree of effort on your part. As you read through them, keep your focus on the results you want to achieve. Also, understand that the benefits of experimenting with these strategies will usually be even greater than what you might imagine. For instance, if you change any limiting beliefs you might have around money and happen to win the lottery, you will be more likely to hold onto your fortune and enjoy it. Beyond becoming a lottery winner, if you decide to set goals around financial prosperity, with the right habits, you won't procrastinate on doing what it takes to turn those goals into reality.

Born into poverty, John Paul DeJoria became one of the wealthiest people in the world by founding dozens of successful businesses, including Paul Mitchell hair products. This is what he says about effort and doing the things that will bring you success.

The difference between successful people and unsuccessful people is that successful people do the things that unsuccessful people don't want to do.

You now have the chance to learn how to do some of the things that have helped successful people make their dreams come true.

We are all unique in our learning styles and the best ways to change our behaviors and habits. That makes this is a situation where one size doesn't fit all, so in this chapter I'm providing a variety of techniques for you to explore. There is no one right way or one right combination of techniques to stop procrastinating. Some techniques work better for some people than others. But you won't know which techniques work for you until you try them out.

Your job is to become like a detective or a private investigator who is looking for clues and trying to solve a crime. In other words, use a **detective mindset.** First, zero in on when your procrastination takes over and steals your time. Then experiment with the techniques and apply them in your life for long enough to give them a fair trial. Give each one you try a whole-hearted, good-faith effort. Write down the ones you test and the results you get. Let your results speak for themselves to help you identify which techniques are a good fit for you.

You will only need to do seven of the following techniques one time to get the benefit. For the others, depending on how long it takes you to get feedback from your own experiences, try each particular technique for about a week. Experimenting with each one for two weeks could be even better. But you should know pretty quickly if a technique will be one you can rely on.

Take your time with each strategy. There's no rush. The skills you develop will be with you for the rest of your life, so it pays to spend enough time with each one. Also, give yourself lots of permission to mess up and make mistakes. Any mistakes you make are a normal part of the learning process, and each mistake has at least one lesson for you to learn about what to do differently the next time. You can come back to this chapter again and again until you learn the strategies that work for you. Sometimes just learning one or two strategies that you use consistently can be enough to help you get past your procrastination and start making progress toward your goals.

When you experiment, I encourage you to regularly assure your Inner Child that as you learn how to stop procrastinating, your Fun One will still get to do the things it enjoys. You can say things like, "I promise I won't ask you to give up your play time. We will still have plenty of time to do the things you like to do. Plus, I'll look for ways you can help me so you can have fun along the way." This type of self-talk will help diminish any sense of seriousness or even dread when you think about getting more focused on your goals. We will cover affirmations later in this chapter, but for now, you can also use affirmations like,

I'm grateful I can finally figure out how to overcome my procrastination and start achieving my goals.

81

My future is suddenly looking brighter!

I suggest you start by doing the first nine activities in order. Most of them don't take that long. Some only take about five minutes, and you only need to do them once. But these nine activities have the potential to help you stop procrastinating immediately, no matter how strong your resistance might be. In fact, some of my students have resolved their problems by simply doing the first strategy that's described.

Next, read through the rest of the activities, then come back and try the ones you are drawn to, the ones that seem most likely to work for you. Keep experimenting with these techniques until you discover the ones that help the most. I experimented with all of these techniques and found the ones that work best for me, but some work better in certain situations than others, so I use them at different times. However, I keep all of them in my toolbox of tips and strategies, ready to go for whenever I hit a snag.

I have grouped these techniques into three categories: before you procrastinate, during the time you are procrastinating, and after you procrastinate. The categories aren't hard and fast. For example, you may find that some of the strategies listed for after you procrastinate work better for you before you get sidetracked. But in general, these categories will guide you as you put on your detective hat and finally figure out what will work for you.

You will need to pick something to focus on as you experiment with the strategies. I call this your **practice goal**. You can choose anything you want. I suggest using the goal you identified in Chapter Two, the one you want to achieve by the time you finish reading this book. If you have already achieved that goal, choose another goal, preferably something you are currently procrastinating on, because that will give you immediate feedback on whether a strategy is working compared to what you have been doing. The next chapter is on goal setting. You can also select a goal using the guidelines in that chapter, then use that goal as you explore the following techniques. Once you complete a goal, pick another one you can use for practice.

Use These Techniques *Before* You Procrastinate

A good place to start is by getting the big picture of the patterns of your procrastination. You have already done that by writing down your procrastination story. Your story is the view from 10,000 feet above your life. Let's drop down a little closer and get more specific details.

1. Ask yourself if you are overcommitted.

Some people think they are procrastinators, when actually they are overcommitted. They are trying to do too much and simply don't have enough hours in the day to do it all. Many of my clients ask for help with time management because they want to get more done. And yet when we explore their current responsibilities and their goals, it becomes obvious they are not being realistic about how much time and energy those take.

Procrastination and overcommitment will often look the same, but they have different solutions. If you're overcommitted, you need to do less in one or more areas of your life. This can be a quick fix and can be accomplished in a number of ways, like delegation. Some people are both procrastinators and overcommitted. They need to address both issues. But for right now, ask yourself, "Am I procrastinating, or am I overcommitted?" If it's overcommitment, you need to cut back.

Related to the issue of overcommitment is **the difference between being busy and being productive,** between doing busywork and getting results. Many people procrastinate on their most important goals by doing day-to-day busywork with things that aren't that important. This busywork doesn't take you any closer to achieving your priorities and the results you want. It simply consumes the time you might have to work on what's most important and makes you *feel* like you're making progress. Often, the busywork feels comfortable and familiar, unlike some of your most important goals which can take you out of your comfort zone and into all kinds of feelings you would rather avoid. When you answer the question, "Am I procrastinating, or am I overcommitted?" also consider whether any overcommitment tasks are low priority, busywork, or avoidance activities that take up your time but don't move you toward where you want to be. If they are, look for ways to either stop doing them altogether or reduce the amount of time you spend on them.

2. Identify your procrastination activities.

Once you either rule out or resolve any overcommitment and busywork issues, then identify the tasks you procrastinate on, what I call your **procrastination activities**. What are the things you put off and either do late or not at all? Make a list of the tasks you avoid most often. For example, do you procrastinate on household chores like cleaning and doing laundry? What about self-care activities like eating healthy foods and getting enough exercise? Do you procrastinate on taking care of your finances, like updating your savings plan? Or do you put off doing things in your relationships, like getting together with friends?

Write down the things you typically avoid. Take five minutes and make your list. Think in terms of major areas of your life: relationships (family and friends), personal growth (like reading this book), job or career, school (if you're a student), finances, health and fitness, household, and the hobbies or recreation you do in your free time.

Procrastination takes two different forms: **comfortable procrastination**, which has no negative consequences, and **problem procrastination**, which causes major or minor negative consequences. I may need to clean my garage, but waiting until later is fine, because a delay won't cause any negative consequences. This is an example of comfortable procrastination. In contrast, if you don't pay your bills on time, you'll get a penalty fee. If you drag your feet when dealing with health issues, they might become a serious problem. These are examples of problem procrastination.

After you have written down the activities you typically avoid, take an extra minute and mark the problem procrastination activities on your list, the ones you need to address right away. When you are selecting which goals you want to focus on, I suggest you consider starting with problem procrastination activities, the ones where waiting can lead to major problems down the road.

3. Write down your avoidance activities.
In a previous chapter you identified your main, go-to avoidance activity, the thing you do most often instead of doing what you should be doing. Take a few minutes to write that down, along with the other activities you use to avoid doing what you should be doing. For example, you might check Twitter, respond to text messages, play online games, get something to eat, watch television, or scroll through your favorite online news sites. These can also be just flat-out **time wasters**, even if you aren't using them

to avoid something you need to get done.

While you're listing your avoidance activities, I encourage you to also list your time wasters—the things you do that add no significant value or enjoyment to your life. These can include social activities like happy hours, partying, and spending time with people who are complainers or who are stuck in their own lives and tend to bring you down.

4. Increase your awareness.

Awareness is the first step to change because **awareness leads to choice**— the choice to continue your behavior or do something different. Many people find that just becoming more aware of what they are putting off and what they are doing instead helps them change their behavior. It allows them to choose a more productive response, one that leads them to the outcomes and results they want.

Pay more attention to your behavior and how you are using your time. When you find yourself doing one of your avoidance activities, ask yourself, "Am I procrastinating?" You may or may not be putting something else off at that moment. But asking this question will help increase your awareness of your patterns of delay.

Another way to increase your awareness is to do a **daily review**. Sometime in the evening, look back at your day and identify any times when you procrastinated. I suggest you write them down. Also, look for patterns in the times you procrastinate. When you add this information to your awareness of what you do when you procrastinate, your avoidance activities, it can give you an advantage to overcome it.

For example, while I was writing this book, I had two major blocks of time each day when I worked on it. One was first thing in the morning during the golden hours. The second was right after lunch. Doing a daily review for only several days helped me see there were two times when I was most likely to get off track. One was right after my morning writing when my brain needed a break. If I wasn't careful, I could go online and spend way too much time in mindless scrolling instead of doing something productive that didn't take much thought, like feeding my pets or preparing part of my breakfast.

I was also more likely to procrastinate by checking emails right after lunch, before I got focused on something I needed to do for the book. Just knowing those were my two most vulnerable times—and knowing my usual avoidance activity was going online—helped me guard against procrastination. The awareness I gained from a daily review made it easier to stay on my schedule and stay focused on my writing, which was my most important priority at the time. It only took a few minutes over a few evenings to figure that out.

5. Notice what you do between tasks.

Part of increasing your awareness is noticing what you do between planned activities. Many procrastinators do fine once they get focused on a task, begin to engage with actually doing the task, and start the flow of dopamine. They tend to drift into distractions and become more vulnerable to procrastinating as they transition between one activity and another, such as waking up, getting ready for the day, going to work, and focusing in on a goal. Knowing in advance that you may be more likely to indulge in one of your avoidance activities during these transition periods can help you stay on track.

That vulnerable transition time is another reason why taking healthy breaks from periods of focus and concentration becomes more important. Unless you're on a roll and working productively, consider taking a break every 45 minutes to an hour, which is when most of us start to lose our focus. These breaks may include the fun activities for your Inner Child that you identified earlier— maybe talking with family and friends, biking or working out, checking your social media accounts, or playing with your children or pets. Activities for shorter breaks may include simply getting up, stretching, walking around, getting a drink of water, or eating a healthy snack. If you want to focus and concentrate after your break, be careful about checking your phone or going online during your break. As you probably already know, that can steal your time and attention for hours.

There are also those times when you need a break from working on your priority goal, but you don't necessarily need a complete break or to stop working on it altogether. It's more like you just need a change of pace by doing something else that is productive but doesn't take as much concentration. Instead of drifting off into one of your avoidance activities, you can take what I call a **productive break**—do something that needs to get done but doesn't take much brain power. After a short break (maybe ten to fifteen minutes), you go back to focusing on your priority. I suggest that you make a list of these activities in advance so you don't have to think of them when you need to use them. For example, you can make a shopping list, clean off part of your desk, take the trash out, or return a phone call. I already mentioned how some busywork activities that work for me are meal preparation or feeding my pets. Without a list of possibilities, you may automatically reach for your phone and start scrolling. Far too many times, that becomes our default time filler if we don't know what else to do.

6. Identify your procrastination triggers.

Another way to increase your awareness is to identify your procrastination triggers. Besides trying to do one of the tasks you usually procrastinate on, (the things that make you feel uncomfortable), what else can trigger your procrastination? Often this is related to your physical or emotional state at the time. For example, it's difficult for any of us to do things we don't want to do when we already feel tired or hungry. And if we are emotionally upset, it can be harder to break through our normal resistance to start an uncomfortable task. If you feel lonely or angry, for instance, those feelings can make it more difficult to do what you should do. In Alcoholics Anonymous (AA) programs, they refer to these four triggers as HALT (hungry, angry, lonely or tired) to help identify times when people might be more likely to relapse and start drinking. Many people also procrastinate when they're upset about a conflict in a relationship. Any of these things can trigger your delays. Sometimes you can push through that resistance, and sometimes it is better to deliberately wait, take care of the trigger situation, and work on your goal when you feel more grounded.

I've found that it rarely works for me to begin a project after dinner when my mind and body want to slow down before going to sleep. It's much better for me to go to bed and get started first thing in the morning. Or if I'm hungry, I usually need to eat something before asking myself to do something that's difficult or emotionally charged. These are examples of **strategic procrastination**, where you consciously choose to wait until a later time, because that will increase your odds of success. **Much of procrastination is about timing—about when you get things done.** With strategic procrastination, you consciously and intentionally decide to change the timing of when you do a task and do it later rather than sooner.

7. Ask your Inner Child what it needs to feel safe.

All of us have remnants of a young child living inside of us. Our beliefs, emotions, and memories keep this little child alive as an active part of our lives, even when we aren't consciously aware of that. When you procrastinate, your Inner Child may be feeling a whole host of emotions, including bored, scared, lost, mad, frustrated, overwhelmed, and helpless. It probably doesn't know how to handle those feelings.

To get started on this activity, pretend you are communicating with your inner four-year-old. First, imagine how you looked at that age—really cute, but maybe unsure, afraid, and not knowing what to do. Looking at an actual picture of yourself when you were that age can be helpful. Then seeing that image in your mind or looking at the picture, ask your Inner Child what it needs in order to feel safe. Give it complete permission to tell you whatever it needs. Don't judge. Don't criticize. Just accept. Write down what your Inner Child tells you. This will bring your internal conflicts into the open so you can start to diffuse your inner power struggle. Here are some examples of what your Inner Child might say:

> I need more sleep.
>
> I need you to quit pushing to do things when I'm already tired.
>
> I need you to talk to me when I get scared and tell me it's okay.
>
> I need healthy food so I'll feel better.
>
> I need more exercise. I don't like feeling this bad. I need to be more active.
>
> I need you to be nice to me and stop saying mean things.
>
> I need to know what you want me to do and for you to praise me after I do it.
>
> I need you to stop ignoring me for so long when you work or when you're on your phone.
>
> I'm just a little kid. I need your love. I need your approval. I need you to help me.

Once you know what your Inner Child needs to feel safe, then give those things to your child. Do everything you can to help your Inner Child feel loved, safe, and secure—not just when you are trying to overcome your procrastination—but all the time. This strategy is recommended by author and speaker Debbie Lynn Grace, who has also found it to be an effective way to work through inner blocks.

Please note that some people don't feel comfortable with Inner Child activities. If that's the case for you, you can still benefit from exercises like this by thinking of your Inner Child as your brain or your subconscious mind. If you ask your brain what it needs, you will usually get many of the same answers as if you were asking your Inner Child.

8. Make a win-win agreement with your Inner Child.

Right now, you may be at an impasse with your Inner Child and your Inner Adult with neither side willing to budge, which means you continue to procrastinate like you always have. One strategy that works well to break through this impasse is to decide what each of your competing parts is willing to do to achieve your goals. Write down specific things your Inner Child and your Inner Adult promise to do so they can both feel happy and safe. This compromise or middle ground needs to be fair to both parties or else it won't work. Here's an example.

Inner Adult Promises:

1. I promise to give you healthy play time every single day.

2. I promise not to mentally beat you up, criticize, or berate you. Period.

3. I promise I won't completely ignore you when I work for long periods of time.

4. I promise to try to make work time also fun, so you can enjoy it along with me (e.g., turn it into a game).

5. I promise to pay more attention to when you feel upset and when that happens, to reassure you with positive and nurturing self-talk.

Inner Child Promises:

1. I promise to not sabotage your plans first thing in the morning.

2. I promise to try to be less impulsive. But you have to help me by moving temptations out of sight, especially your phone.

3. I promise I won't get so scared when you break the safety rules we have always lived by—as long as you keep reassuring me that it's okay. Go slow at first so I have a chance to get used to something new.

After you have written down the agreement, I suggest you date it and keep it someplace where you will see it often. If you can get a commitment or buy-in from the two parts of yourself on this kind of a compromise, it will help you avoid the standoffs that have kept you so stuck in the past. Plus, you can turn your Inner Adult promises into specific goals and deliberately choose to achieve them. Probably without knowing it, most highly successful people have learned to create win-win situations for their Inner Child and their Inner Adult. They usually work hard and play hard. Now you know how to do the same. Again, you can make this agreement between your Inner Adult and your brain or subconscious mind if that's more comfortable for you.

9. Use the Four-step Peace Process

I encourage you to learn this four-step method early on as you experiment with these strategies. You can use it before, during and after you procrastinate. It has enormous potential to break through your inner blocks and help you move forward quickly and easily. Part of why it works so well is because it is a **mind-body technique**. It addresses what happens in your mind—and in your body—that causes you to procrastinate.

The underlying basis for this strategy is included in several books, *Power vs. Force* and *Letting Go*, by the late David Hawkins. As a psychiatrist, Hawkins became an internationally known speaker on consciousness research and had one of the most successful psychiatric therapy practices in the U.S. People came from all over the world to get his help. The woman who wrote the foreword to *Letting Go* said that just by reading Hawkins' material, an addiction she'd had for many years went away, her anxiety disorder no longer bothered her, and long-standing fears and resentments simply disappeared. She also said that as of the time of her writing, her changes had lasted and seemed to be permanent. That's how powerful the strategy can be. I've heard similar stories over and over from other people who have learned a specific version of this technique from my life coach, Christian Mickelsen, which is why I so enthusiastically recommend it. Later on, I'll explain more about why it works. But for now, follow along with these four steps.

Step 1. Pay Attention. Think of one thing you are currently procrastinating on, one task where you feel stuck right now. Now think about actually doing the task you want to do. How do you feel about doing whatever it will take to get the task done? Identify the emotion that makes you feel by giving it a name. Is it fear? Dread? Anxiety? Anger? Frustration? If you don't know exactly what you're feeling, that's okay. It can be helpful to name the feeling, but it's not necessary. Some people can't identify exactly what emotion they are feeling, but they definitely know it's not pleasant.

Step 2. Find the Feeling. Most procrastination is about avoiding unpleasant emotions. One of the reasons this technique works so well is because our negative emotions often get trapped in our bodies and create emotional blocks. So using a mind-body technique like the Peace Process makes sense. After you have identified the emotion you are feeling as best you can, then look for where in your body you feel that emotion. In this step, you are simply finding where in your body the uncomfortable feeling is located.

Quickly scan your body with your inner awareness, from the top of your head to the bottoms of your feet. Identify where in your body you feel that emotion, which you may experience as tightness, tension or discomfort. Sometimes it may feel like it's in your chest or stomach, or maybe your neck or shoulders. Some people experience the feeling in their head. There's no right or wrong here. Go with your first impression. If you can't locate the feeling, then guess where it would be.

Next, put one finger on the place where the emotion feels the most intense. Guess if you need to. The emotion may move around and go to different parts of your body. It can also change into a different emotion. Your job is to simply notice where you feel the feeling and continue to put one finger on where it's the most intense. If the feeling moves to another part of your body, move your finger along with it. If you feel the emotion somewhere on your back and can't reach it, put your finger on the front of your body, in the location that corresponds to that place on your back. Then ask yourself, "On a scale of one to ten, how intense is this feeling?" One is the least intense and ten is the most intense. Give the intensity a number within this range.

Step 3. Observe the Feeling. As you continue to focus on this place in your body, notice if the feeling seems to be changing or moving. Is it swirling, pulsating, getting bigger, getting smaller, getting more or less intense? Then stay with the feeling and simply observe the part of your body where you experience the feeling as the most intense. **Do not try to make the feeling go away.** Don't analyze it. Don't try to understand it. And don't try to change it. Instead, in your thoughts, send this part of your body acceptance. Send it compassion. And if you can, send it love. You have probably spent years trying to avoid this emotion, just wanting to get rid of it. But the goal is to accept the feeling exactly the way it is right now. No judgement. Just acceptance. Allow it to be whatever it wants to be. Allow it to do whatever it wants to do, and to go wherever it wants to go in your body.

If you find yourself thinking about the story behind that feeling, bring your awareness back to simply observing the place in your body where you feel the emotion the most intensely. In other words, stay out of your head, and just observe the feeling in your body, sending it acceptance, compassion, and love. Give it complete permission to be and do whatever it wants.

We usually reject parts of ourselves we don't like, which creates more blocks. Through our thoughts, we keep repeating the story behind the feeling, which keeps the story alive and the emotion stuck inside of us. Love heals. Acceptance frees us. Our focused awareness and attention act like a laser beam shining a light into the exact spot where the emotional block is the most intense. That attention—along with our compassion—help to dissolve and release the block so energy can once again flow freely through that part of our bodies. It's like a stream that has temporarily gotten dammed up with a log jam. The logs finally break apart and the stream can start to flow freely again.

Step 4. Act. Continue observing the feeling until the intensity level reaches a zero or a one. If there seem to be places in your body where you still feel the emotion, repeat Steps Two and Three. When the intensity has dissipated, you will usually feel either peaceful or more of a neutral feeling. But the emotion you have been avoiding will often be released. To test this out, again think of actually doing the task you have been procrastinating on. If that feeling remains a zero or a one, you have successfully used the Peace Process to help release an emotion and the block that has caused you to procrastinate on that task.

If what you've been procrastinating on is the kind of task you can do for a short time right now, I suggest that you *act* on your task by doing it for at least five minutes. Maybe longer if that feels right. Actually doing the task is the final test as to whether your emotional block has been released. Also, doing the task you have been avoiding will give you a sense of success and confidence that you can get back on track after procrastination interrupts your plans. It's similar to immediately getting back on a horse after you have fallen off. You want to end up with a sense of mastery over your fear or any other emotions that might get in your way. If the emotion gets triggered while you are doing the task—either now or later—simply repeat this Peace Process until you are completely free from any internal resistance.

Once you learn the steps, getting to peace with an intensity level of zero or one can take less time, sometimes just minutes. Some of our emotional blocks take longer to release than others. That means you may need to keep repeating this four-step method until the blocks are dissolved. For example, I had a block in my stomach area that required lots of love and attention and going through these steps multiple times. But because that block was related to my procrastination, dissolving that particular block put me on the fast track to completing my goals. I had absolutely no desire to stall or mess around. Poof. Just like that, whatever had been holding me back was gone.

Benefits of the Peace Process

One of the things that can be so appealing about this technique is that it isn't a cathartic method of expressing emotions like crying, beating a pillow, or talking about your feelings with someone else. It doesn't involve any of the "touchy-feely" techniques of emotional expression that so many people feel uncomfortable with and want to avoid. Instead, once you identify the feeling or the place in your body where you feel stuck, you focus on the physical sensation of that feeling in your body and just concentrate on the most intense spot. Often, people who are doing the Peace Process will spontaneously close their eyes to increase their concentration. They look like they are meditating or simply concentrating intently. Almost always, they are calm and focused within. Occasionally people will cry, and that's okay. But usually their crying means they are thinking about the story associated with the feeling. When they focus on their body instead of their thoughts about their story, their crying usually stops.

I learned the specific steps of this strategy when I went through the coaching certification training offered by my coach, Christian Mickelsen, who is a bestselling author and trainer to life coaches, business coaches, and other types of coaches around the world. Then I adapted it to apply specifically to procrastination, as I have just described.

Mickelsen calls it the **Peace Process**, and he has been teaching it for about the past fifteen years to help people resolve all kinds of issues, including procrastination. His book, *Abundance Unleashed*, describes the many ways he helps people. Mickelsen believes the Peace Process is one of the fastest ways to help people get unstuck and achieve their goals. Having worked for decades as a personal counselor, with certain exceptions, I agree. Some people need to get into more traditional counseling and therapy because of the issues they are dealing with. I will cover some of these issues in later chapters. But I wish I had known about the Peace Process when I was doing so much one-on-one counseling. I could have used this technique to help many of my clients resolve their issues in hours instead of weeks or months. I have since learned that for many people, overcoming procrastination is one of those issues where the Peace Process works well. Plus, you don't need a counselor or therapist to help you with this method. Once you learn how, you can use the technique with yourself, which means there's no cost involved. It's free to anyone who wants to use it.

Doing this four-step method has changed me in ways that expressing my emotions never did. For example, as soon as I got home from my certification training where we did the Peace Process a lot, a feral cat I had been feeding for years suddenly wanted me to pet her. Before that, she wouldn't come any closer than six feet from me. After the training, I felt noticeably more at peace in general, and I think the cat could feel that peacefulness within me.

I was so excited about sharing this process that I scheduled times to meet with friends, family, and colleagues so I could teach it to them. Overwhelmingly, they found it helpful. They also noticed the changes in me. As one friend said, "You seem so calm." I was, and for the most part, still am. And so far, the changes in me have lasted. The same goes for the coaching clients I've taught it to. One client was able to release the emotions that were underneath her debilitating post-traumatic stress disorder (PTSD), all within a matter of several hours. As of this writing, she hasn't had any more problems.

Using the Peace Process with My Procrastination

I vividly remember the first time I used this technique with my own procrastination. I needed to sort through a stack of paperwork that was about two feet tall. Because of what it contained, I had to look at every single piece of paper and make a decision about what to do with it. Ugh. I dreaded it. I was sitting in my office at the time. My computer was already turned on. Out of the blue, the thought crossed my mind that I could hop online and catch up on the news first and do the sorting later. I immediately saw that Sneaky was trying to lure me away from what I needed to do, and I urgently yelled out loud, "Peace Process! Peace Process!"

In that awareness, I sat in my office, found the feeling of dread that was in my abdomen, identified the intensity as a seven, then sent it acceptance and love. It didn't take more than ten minutes for the feeling to dissolve. At that point, I felt completely at peace about sorting through the paperwork, and I was able to get it done quickly and easily, almost as if it took no effort—*because I had no internal resistance*. Afterward I felt ecstatic, so pleased with myself, and absolutely thrilled because I could see the opportunities that would open up in my life by using this one simple technique.

What's even more phenomenal about this method is that **it can eliminate limiting beliefs—without having to know what they are**. In *Letting Go*, Hawkins says that one feeling can create thousands of associated thoughts. For example, people who were abused as children often think about that abuse thousands of times after it happens. The Peace Process provides a way to release the underlying painful feeling of that abuse, along with the associated thoughts that have accumulated over what could be years.

I felt a seismic shift in my brain when I understood that a feeling can create limiting thoughts and hold those thoughts in place. In all my decades of studying counseling and psychology, I had never heard that. Instead, the recommended process was always to identify the limiting thoughts first, then work like crazy to change them to something more positive—usually through insight and lots and lots of repetition—using positive affirmations and other strategies. After that, the emotions associated with them would usually start to go away. But no, Hawkins was saying to release the emotion first, and the disempowering thoughts will naturally and automatically disappear. Wow. That is a game changer.

Before I learned this process, I had always been the kind of person who wanted to know what I was thinking, because that gave me a sense of control. Plus, I thought I *had* to know what my limiting beliefs were in order to change them. But this process bypassed my need for control and helped me change my beliefs without knowing exactly what they were. What's interesting is that usually within a couple of days of doing this technique, the main limiting beliefs that had been released will somehow drift into my awareness, so eventually, I do know what they were. Many people who work with this method also have the same experience. It makes the process of changing these beliefs so much simpler and faster.

This technique can work when you are stuck or emotionally upset about anything. For instance, if you're angry at your parents for teaching you limiting beliefs, you can do the Peace Process around that anger and let it go. If you feel guilty about all the times you've procrastinated in the past, you can release your guilt. When you feel scared about doing something in the future that is outside your comfort zone, determine if there's any real danger, and if not, let go of that fear so you can move forward with calmness and a clear mind.

Once you learn how to do the Peace Process with yourself, you can also use it with other people. Even people who are just starting to use this technique often find that it helps the person they are working with, and they are eager to teach it to their children. You don't have wait until you think you can do it perfectly. Plus, someone who has learned the technique but isn't a therapist can facilitate it for you. If you want to read Mickelsen's description of the Peace Process, it's in *Abundance Unleashed.*

I want to be clear that I'm not suggesting that you always try to make all your negative emotions simply go away. Instead, I believe all our emotions are gifts. The pleasant and the unpleasant ones. The comfortable and the uncomfortable ones. Together with our thoughts and intuition, they form this exquisite internal GPS system that can guide us through life. Emotions like fear can keep us safe and protect us from harm. Emotions like anger can alert us when we've been mistreated. Sadness helps us recognize and grieve our losses. Our positive emotions bring us hope and joy, gratitude and peace. Life without emotions feels empty.

However, the vast majority of us aren't taught how to deal with our emotions in healthy ways. Instead, whenever any emotion makes us feel uncomfortable, we often try to make it go away before accepting the gift of its message. We try to ignore it. Deny it's there. Distract ourselves with things like our phones. Stuff it down with food. Turn to addictions like alcohol and drugs. In short, we numb. But one of the problems is that **we can't numb our emotions selectively**. To the extent that we numb any one emotion, we numb them all. To the extent that we numb our pain, we also numb our joy.

Because so few people know healthy ways to express their emotions, I described nine techniques for healthy emotional expression in my first book, *The Power of Life Lessons*. However, even *after* people express their emotions in healthy ways, sometimes they are still left with what I call an **emotional residue**, where some of those emotions remain inside their bodies and can cause problems in their lives. The Peace Process and other mind-body techniques can help release these remaining feelings so that emotional residue doesn't keep people stuck. I discuss this more in detail in Chapter Seven on healthy habits.

To sum up this section, these first nine activities I just described may be effective enough for you to release your limiting beliefs and stop procrastinating. However, many of us may still need additional efforts to change our unproductive habits, the ones that are deeply engrained in our behavior, the ones we do automatically without thinking. This next section provides more strategies to help you get back on track—after you have already fallen into the procrastination trap.

Use These Techniques *During* Your Procrastination

In the last chapter, I described how the famous football quarterback Joe Namath quit drinking. He was able to stop by giving a name to the thoughts that told him to drink. There was a reason he chose Slick as the name for that inner voice. Namath knew he was procrastinating by not quitting altogether, but Slick could fool him into drinking by saying things like, "It's okay. Just this one time." I call my procrastination Sneaky for the same reason—that your procrastination can be incredibly creative, quick, and clever. It knows how to dupe you. It knows what you will fall for. It sabotages your willpower and manipulates your reasoning with excuses that sound perfectly rational at the time.

We can all get triggered into impulsive reactions in a split second. That's why it is important to develop enough awareness that you can recognize when you are stalling as it is happening. Eliminating the underlying beliefs that have kept you procrastinating is a first step. You now know how to do that by using the Peace Process; I describe additional techniques like affirmations later in this chapter. But you may still be left with your impulsive habits of putting things off. Breaking those habits often requires more experimenting.

In this phase of overcoming your procrastination, awareness is the key to giving yourself a choice, the choice to do something different, to do something productive instead of procrastinating. Sometimes you can't catch your procrastination soon enough. You suddenly realize that your time thief pulled a fast one and you've ended up checking your phone without consciously realizing that was happening.

The following activities will help you become aware of your procrastination in the moment, as it is playing out. Watch yourself. Observe your own behavior. Be especially vigilant when you are trying to do something you typically procrastinate on and when you are doing one of your avoidance activities, the things you use as stall tactics. As you read through these techniques, keep this question in mind, **"Which ones of these seem like they might work for me?"**

10. Breathe. Move your body.

When you find yourself procrastinating, stop doing your avoidance activity and simply breathe. Take a few deep, conscious breaths to break the pattern. By deliberately deciding to do something like deep breathing, you take your mental focus out of your impulsive limbic system and into your prefrontal cortex, where you have a better chance of using your willpower to change your thoughts and behavior. I've found that breathing is the quickest way to get unstuck, but any kind of physical movement can have the same effect. For example, do a few jumping jacks or take a short walk, even it's just around your house or office. In fact, simply smiling can do wonders to lift your mood and help you get unstuck (Google this and see what a surprising difference it can make). Our bodies can help change our beliefs by influencing how we think and feel about ourselves. As Tony Robbins says, "If you want to change your psychology, first change your physiology."

Amy Cuddy, a social psychologist at Harvard, did some fascinating research on this topic. She found that when people changed their body position and assumed what she calls a **power pose** for only two minutes, they felt more powerful and confident. It even changed their body chemistry (their testosterone increased by 28 percent). In general, this pose means making your body more open and expansive and taking up more space. For example, either sitting or standing, stretch your arms out away from your body, put your shoulders back, and keep your feet apart. Cuddy describes how one of her students was failing her class, didn't feel like she belonged at Harvard, and wanted to drop out of school. Cuddy taught the her how to do the power pose, and even though the student felt like a fake in the beginning, she kept doing it and eventually became more confident and assertive. The student ended up graduating. She didn't just fake it until she made it. **She faked it until she became it.**

This technique is easy, quick, and free. I encourage you to learn and practice it before you need it, like right before you give a talk, before a job interview, or when you get bogged down by procrastination. I've started taking a power pose before I speak to a group of people. I'm usually seated right before I talk, and all I need to do is take a few deep breaths, put my chin up, uncross my legs, and stretch my arms out behind my chair for several minutes. I've been amazed at how something this simple can make such a big difference in my level of self-confidence. I encourage you to learn how to do this by watching Cuddy's twenty-minute TED Talk called

"Your Body Language May Shape Who You Are" (see ted.com/speakers/ amy_cuddy). Like with her student, it could change your life.

11. Ask yourself, "What just happened?"

Once you realize you are procrastinating, stop whatever you are doing, take a mental step back from that moment, and ask yourself, "What just happened?" Put on your detective hat. Become intensely curious and determined to discover what triggered your procrastination. Backtrack in your thoughts and try to figure out what you were feeling and what you were thinking that caused you to abandon your plans. You may not be able to identify the emotions or the thoughts. That's okay. Just become more aware of when your behavior changed from moving toward your goal to moving away from it.

Let's say you find yourself on TikTok when you never planned to open it up. Click out and ask, "What just happened?" Remember what you had originally set out to do. Maybe you planned to clean out your inbox of old email messages. Maybe you never intended to go online in the first place but to change into your workout clothes and head to the gym. Look for the emotion and thoughts that triggered you to open TikTok instead. Finding the exact trigger point that caused you to start procrastinating may be enough for you to re-focus your attention on your original plans.

However, if you still feel stuck, you can use the four-step Peace Process. Take a moment to find where in your body you feel emotionally stuck, put your finger on the most intense place, ask yourself how intense the feeling is on a scale of zero to ten, and send it love and acceptance. Do this until the intensity level reaches a zero or one and you are left feeling either neutral or at peace. You can also use other strategies in this chapter, including the next strategy, to become more aware of what triggered your avoidance.

12. Write down your thoughts and feelings.

Remember, at least 80 percent of what slows you down or stops you from achieving your goals is the Inner Game, the mindset, the thoughts and emotions that create your internal blocks. In this strategy, you piggyback on the awareness that comes from asking, "What just happened?" and write down any thoughts or emotions you become aware of when you tried to get something done but couldn't. What were you thinking when that happened? What were you feeling? Write down both of those. Here are some examples.

- *I don't want to go to the gym. I'm tired, and it takes too much energy.*

I'll just watch a little TV instead. Besides, I can make up for it by going to the gym an extra time later this week.

- *Working on that report is frustrating. I don't know how to write it. I'll just check Instagram really fast, then I'll work on the report.*

- *I'm so mad at myself for eating those cookies and getting off my diet. But since I've already blown it for today, I might as well eat the last two cookies and finish off the bag. I'll get back on my diet tomorrow, and then I'll be extra strict about what I eat.*

The more you increase your awareness, the better you will get at catching those thoughts and feelings as they happen. That will start to give you more choice about whether or not you procrastinate. You will understand that they are just thoughts, not mandates, and you can choose to do something else. You can choose to follow through with your goals instead of taking the well-worn path of falling into immediate gratification.

Eventually those kinds of thoughts will set off an alarm in your head that your procrastination is getting ready to rob you of your goals. Your procrastination can sound so logical at the time, but make no mistake about it. You are getting conned. You're getting sweet-talked and hoodwinked into giving up the goals that are important to you. As you keep watching and observing, you will learn how to recognize the con job as it is happening.

Sometimes just getting the competing thoughts and feelings out of your head and into writing is enough for you to get past them. You may realize those thoughts and feelings came from limiting beliefs you used to believe but don't anymore, and you're simply acting out of habit. In that case, you may be able to continue working on your goal. However, if you write them down and still can't move forward, you can use additional strategies from this chapter to get unstuck, including affirmations.

13. Use positive affirmations.

Once you have identified the thoughts that are behind your procrastination, you can use positive affirmations to help steer your behavior into productive activities instead. First, write down the procrastination thoughts, then make up empowering statements to counteract them. Here are some examples.

- Procrastination thought: *I don't want to do this right now.*
  Instead affirm: *This won't be any easier later on. I might as well start and at least get some of it done now.*

- Procrastination thought: *I can't get anything done when I feel this overwhelmed.*
  Instead affirm: *It's okay to feel overwhelmed. I don't have to run away from that feeling. Instead, I'll use the Peace Process and release it so I can work on my goal.*

Continue to monitor your thoughts, and when you notice the ones that are causing you to procrastinate, immediately think of an empowering statement, write it down, and say it out loud. As we covered earlier, usually the most recent voice in your head that is the one that causes you to act in a certain way. Don't let your voice of procrastination have the last word.

If you know the limiting beliefs that are underneath your procrastination, write those down as well. Then challenge them. Are they even true? Maybe they were true when you were a child, but now they don't match who you are as an adult. Look for factual evidence that your limiting beliefs may not be ironclad, hard-and-fast, true-every-time statements. Then make up empowering statements that are a more accurate reflection of the person you are today. Here are a few examples.

- Limiting belief: *That's too hard. I can't do something that difficult.*
  Empowering statement: *What I know about myself is that if I keep working on something, and if I focus on it for long enough, I'll eventually figure it out.*

- Limiting belief: *Something bad will happen if I go after my big goals. Those are way too scary.*
  Empowering statement: *Now I understand how moving out of my comfort zone is frightening. But I can learn how to do that and still stay safe. Plus, I know I'll regret it if I don't at least try to achieve my goals.*

- Limiting belief: *I don't deserve to succeed.*
  Empowering statement: *Deep down inside, I know I'm worthy of success, especially if I work hard and give it everything I've got.*

In addition to empowering statements and affirmations that directly address your limiting beliefs, you can also make up general affirmations around your procrastination. I suggest you keep all of your affirmations where you will see them often—on your phone, taped on your bathroom mirror, above your desk. And read them often. Silently and out loud. The point is to constantly expose yourself to affirming messages, and you can gradually start to re-program your subconscious mind. Examples of general affirmations include,

- I'm so thankful I have the time and energy to achieve my goals.
- I'm now aware of how my procrastination tries to trick me.
- I am strong enough to accomplish my goals.
- It's fun to be successful.

Here's one final way to use affirmations. When I was doing my training to become certified as a hypnotherapist, I learned about hypnotic suggestions that are based on what is called **paradoxical intention**. This is where you suggest to yourself that the more the obstacles along your path increase, the more capable you are of handling them and reaching your goal. The hypnotic suggestions worked so well that I started using them as affirmations. And I love them. Here are a few examples.

- The more stress I experience, the more calm, focused, and productive I become.
- The harder it gets to achieve my goals, the more determined I become to succeed.
- The more fear I feel about leaving my comfort zone, the more I dig deep inside and find the courage to face it.

I suggest that you make up your own affirmations based on paradoxical intention in the areas of your life where you feel the most stuck. They will help you become more aware of your obstacles and your response to those obstacles. They work especially well when you are trying to persuade yourself to do things that make you feel anxious and afraid.

I'd like to share two stories that demonstrate how your thoughts determine your behavior. One of my university counseling clients, Ashley, struggled with low self-esteem. Her underlying limiting belief was that *I'm not good enough.* Ashley focused on what she saw as her flaws and weaknesses. She would only remember the times when she felt inadequate and would often take other people's positive comments about her the wrong way.

Ashley was a high achiever, successful in many areas of her life. But no matter how much success she achieved, and regardless of how many people expressed their admiration, respect, or affection, she still saw herself as a failure, as less than. She clung to her thoughts despite tons of feedback to the contrary. In other words, she continued to think and believe that she was inferior, and her thoughts about herself created what she experienced as reality.

I could only work with Ashley for a short time. But during that time, she was able to understand how she learned her limiting beliefs as a young child, and those subconscious scripts kept repeating in every experience in her life, telling her that she was inferior. I taught Ashley about affirmations and how to validate herself by giving herself credit for her many accomplishments. I didn't know about the Peace Process at the time, but I would have also taught her how to use that to help transform her limiting beliefs, without having to know what they were.

Sometimes I still think about Ashley. I wonder how she's doing and wish her well in her life. Even in her early twenties, Ashley seemed highly motivated to improve her life. I'm hoping that motivation helped take her where she wanted to go, and that she's happy and fulfilled.

Contrast Ashley's story to that of Valarie Allman who won the gold medal in discus throwing at the 2020 Olympics in Tokyo. Allman started throwing the discus in her freshman year in high school. She quickly developed her skills and started winning competitions. When she was competing in college, she set her sights on the Olympics. Allman realized that chasing her big dream would require excellent coaching and an increasing focus on her mental game. Her coach suggested that she use affirmations to calm her nerves and increase her self-confidence, affirmations like, "I know I can win. I *will* win."

At first, Allman didn't believe the affirmations and felt awkward saying them. But she kept repeating them for a month, until she felt genuinely convinced they were true. Her beliefs then became her reality. If you're willing to put in the time and effort, affirmations can lead to your own version of Olympic gold. Tell yourself, "I am strong enough to overcome whatever problems come my way. I deserve to be successful. I will succeed." Say those kinds of things to yourself regularly. Out loud. With all the emotion you can muster.

14. Talk to your procrastination. Out loud.
Transforming your limiting thoughts and beliefs helps you become more aware of your procrastination. Another good way to increase your awareness is by magnifying your behavior to make it more obvious. Talking out loud about your procrastination as you are doing it is one of the ways you can magnify it. If you haven't already, give your procrastination a name. Then talk to your procrastination by using the name you gave it. For example, here's what I sometimes say, "Sneaky. No. Not now." Be

firm, like you mean it. Remember why your goal is important to you and use that sense of importance to set boundaries around the time you need to achieve it. More details about this suggestion are included in Chapter Four on Outsmart Impulsiveness.

At times, instead of setting firm boundaries, you may need to talk to your Inner Child with more nurturance and understanding. Here, you're trying to help you Inner Child feel safe and be more cooperative. This may be especially important when you are stepping outside your comfort zone. You can say something like, "I know I'm doing things I've never done before. It's okay to be scared, but you're fine. I will keep you safe. This will end up being a good thing. You'll see."

A variation of this technique is to use **distraction,** which works well for most young children. As an example of using distraction, when your Inner Child wants to play with your cell phone, you can say something like, "Oh, look over here. Here's something we can do right now. Let's see how fast we can clean the kitchen. We'll both feel so much better when that's done." Then immediately start into the cleaning. I sometimes call this a lateral shift. Your Inner Child was focused on your phone. If you shift its attention to another activity that you want to get done like cleaning, many times your child will go along with you, at least for a few minutes, which is usually long enough to start making progress, release some dopamine, and forget about the phone.

I learned about distraction during my first job out of college. As a psychology major, after I graduated the only job I could find was with a daycare center where I was put in charge of a room full of two-year-olds. Thirteen of them, with only one aid to help me out. Oh, boy. Needless to say, it was a challenge. Every morning when the parents dropped them off, many of the toddlers would go into a full-blown meltdown, crying and screaming while clinging to their parents like their lives depended on it. I understood they were experiencing the separation anxiety that is so common at that age, and my heart went out to them. But I still needed to manage the situation.

I quickly learned that I could show them a toy, usually away from the door where the parents had just been, and sometimes within seconds, the children would get focused on the toy and the meltdown would be over. It amazed me how that simple distraction worked almost every time. That's what I'm suggesting you do with you own Inner Child. Use distraction to help it get focused on whatever you as the adult want to do.

15. Promise your Inner Child a reward for good behavior.

Although this strategy may seem more like a bribe, promising a reward for good behavior often works, partly because it assures the child that you're not going to make it wait forever to do something it enjoys. It gives your Inner Child something to look forward to in the near future. Now that you know what your Inner Child enjoys, you can promise it a reward—later in the day—and after your Inner Adult has had time to complete its goal. For example, you might say something like, "I just need to finish this one project. I promise that after that we'll take the dogs for a walk."

16. Set a five-minute goal.

Usually, the hardest part of any task you procrastinate on is getting started. You may be able to persuade your Inner Child into starting by setting a goal to work on whatever you want to get done for just five minutes. That's it. That's all you need to do. However, once you finish five minutes, if you want, you can set another five-minute goal to work on your task. By the time you have been focused on your goal for five to ten minutes, it is usually pretty easy to keep going. I think of this technique as sliding into an easy start.

One time I set a goal to start swimming once a week. I joined a masters swim club so I could use the outdoor pool at a local junior high school. The pool was heated, but especially in the middle of winter, the water would get too cold and it was hard to make myself dive in. So I set a five-minute goal. I promised myself that I would swim two laps, which took me about five minutes, and that if I wanted to get out of the pool and go home after that I could. But over the three years I swam in that pool, I never once cut my workout short. Five minutes was all it took for me to get past my resistance and into the feel-good results from my swim. You can do the same thing with most other types of exercise and tasks.

17. Just show up.

If you can't get yourself to do five minutes, then just show up where you need to be. Take a tiny step toward working on your goal. You don't need to do anything except physically place yourself in the location where you need to be to get something done. For example, you might sit down in front of your computer. You may find that since you're already there, you might as well start your computer. Then you might as well open the file you need to work on. You might as well read just one page of the document you need to finish. Once you're already reading the document, you might as well think about what else you need to do to finish your task. No demands. No reprimands. Just gently coaching yourself into more engagement with your task until your concentration gets stronger, the learning begins to happen, and the dopamine gets going.

18. Use the Peace Process.
This is one of my standard, go-to techniques for before, during and after I procrastinate. I love the fact that by focusing on the emotion that is stuck in my body, I can release lots of limiting beliefs—sometimes in just a few minutes. I encourage you to use it alone or in combination with any of these other techniques.

Here's just one example. About 250 people attended Mickelsen's coaching training where I learned this technique, which was held at a hotel in San Diego. During the training and right after a short break, one of the participants came back into the hotel conference room and asked if he could speak. With a microphone in his hand, he told the rest of us about how he was a real estate agent and that during our break, he had spoken with a client over the phone. This woman was considering a large land purchase but was upset about closing the deal, especially since she and her husband didn't see eye to eye on the purchase.

The agent thought this would be a perfect opportunity to use what he had just learned, so he asked her, "Would you like to feel less upset about this?"

She eagerly replied, "Yes."

He then asked, "Where in your body do you feel that upset feeling?" After she responded, he told her, "Focus on that part of your body. Don't think about why you are upset. Just keep your attention on where in your body you feel upset."

It only took several minutes for her feeling to dissipate, and the woman quickly went into a place of peace. This peaceful feeling calmed her mind, allowed her to think clearly, and she immediately knew she wanted to move forward with the closing. Her final comment to the agent was, "I haven't felt this calm in months."

For all of us there at the conference, this was living proof that the technique could work quickly and effectively for those struggling to make clear-headed decisions.

People who use this technique also find that the energy they've been using to keep a lid on the emotions trapped in their bodies gets released, along with the emotions and beliefs that have kept them stuck. When this energy is no longer being using to suppress emotions, it gets freed up and becomes available to help you achieve your goals and enjoy your life. This boost in energy is a welcomed—and appreciated—extra benefit from using the strategy. I encourage you to practice this technique several times, enough that you remember the steps and find it easy to go through them.

Use These Techniques *After* You Procrastinate

Despite your best efforts, sometimes you won't realize you have procrastinated until after the fact. You look up at the clock and realize 40 minutes have gone by while you did some online shopping, even though you had every intention of working on your priority. That's okay. The following activities will help you get back on track. Experiment with these and find the ones that work best for you.

19. Reschedule a time to work on your goal.
When you procrastinate during the time you had planned to work on a goal, please don't criticize yourself or put yourself down. Instead, see it as an opportunity to learn an important lesson. When it happens, get back on the horse and focus on your goal for at least five minutes, which was described earlier in the fourth step of the Peace Process. This will leave you feeling at least a little more successful and self-confident. If you don't have time right then to focus for even five minutes, then decide exactly when you will work on your goal by scheduling a specific time in your calendar. Write it down. Mark off a time slot. This type of deliberate and intentional scheduling is more likely to lead to success, because next time you will have more awareness of how your inner time thief is likely to sabotage your goal. It's like the saving grace of second chances.

20. Make a not-to-do list.
Once you develop more awareness about your procrastination patterns, you start to see when, where and how you become vulnerable to getting off track. You already know *how* you avoid doing what you should be doing. You avoid it by doing one of your avoidance activities, the time wasters that take you far, far away from your goals. The tricky part is that

sometimes your most enjoyable time wasters can be used as rewards for getting something done. It's all a matter of timing. Do you enjoy your avoidance activity before you work on your goal, or afterward? This relates to Strategy Fifteen that we covered before on rewarding your Inner Child for good behavior.

For example, I rescue animals. New animal rescue videos are constantly posted on YouTube, and they are usually inspiring, heartwarming stories. When I'm watching those as an avoidance activity, Sneaky can justify some of my viewing because I sometimes learn rescue tips that help me get better at it. I can also watch the videos as a reward after doing something I didn't want to do. In other words, whether YouTube is an avoidance activity or a reward is a matter of timing. But YouTube is definitely on my not-to-do list when I want to work on a goal.

21. Ask your Future Self for advice.

This strategy will help you tap into your intuition, your gut hunches, the still small voice within that can provide the perfect solutions to many of your problems. Take about 15 minutes to be alone and have a pen and paper available so you can do some writing. First, sit quietly in a comfortable position, close your eyes, and take a few slow, deep breaths. On each exhale, imagine that you are letting go of any stress, worry, or tension. Keep breathing like this until you feel completely relaxed.

Now imagine that you can communicate with your **Future Self**, when you are eight-five years old. Imagine that your Future Self has lived an extraordinary life and found all the success you ever wanted, including a deep inner sense of peace and joy. When you feel ready, ask your Future Self to give you advice on how to stop procrastinating, on how to keep procrastination from stealing your goals and dreams. What would your Future Self tell you to do? What wisdom would your Future Self share so that you could get past any obstacles you now feel are in your way? Sit quietly and just listen until your Future Self has told you everything you need to hear. Do not judge or question the advice. Just listen and accept.

When your Future Self has finished passing on its wisdom, thank it for all it has shared. Then open your eyes and take as long as you need to write down the advice you were given. Again, this is not the time to question the advice, just get it down on paper. Information that comes from our intuition can quickly fade from memory, so it's important to write it down immediately.

Most people find this activity surprisingly helpful in several ways. They usually get advice that is tailor-made for their particular stumbling blocks. It is practical and gives them concrete, step-by-step instructions on what to do. Many people also find that communicating with their wise Future Self gives them a sense of trust, confidence, and courage. They feel inspired and more motivated to continue with their efforts to finally get past their procrastination and start living their best life.

This strategy can be a tremendous tool to use whenever you get stuck or feel unsure about what to do, not just with procrastination, but with anything in your life. All you need to do is ask your Future Self about that particular situation. Journaling by itself can be a powerful technique to get clarity and inner advice. More information about the benefits of journaling is included in Chapter Seven on healthy habits.

22. Use the Peace Process

As I have mentioned, this process is the fastest way I have found for releasing the mental and emotional blocks that keep us stuck. It is quite astounding when you realize that it can so quickly release life-long patterns of self-sabotage. Once you start using it more regularly, it starts to become more natural and automatic. Here's a shortcut to remember what to do with the feeling that's trapped in your body:

Find it. Feel it. Observe it. Release it.

In preparation for writing this book, I did an in-depth literature review over several years by reading books, journal articles, and online information—anything I could find on how to overcome procrastination. In all my research, I only found a handful of other authors who mention using techniques that involve mind-body work to get past our unnecessary delays. For example, some authors use a technique called Tapping, which is also known as the Emotional Freedom Technique (EFT). The primary authors I found, though, were Christian Mickelsen with the Peace Process, and Nils Salzgeber.

In his book *Stop Procrastinating*, Salzgeber describes his life as a chronic procrastinator. He would get up in the morning, planning to do a healthy morning routine then work on his online business. But instead, he would distract himself by watching television or YouTube videos or by playing video games. His distractions kept him from feeling guilty at the time, but after that he would mentally beat himself with thoughts like *Why can't*

I just sit down and do the things I should do? Why am I so terrible at this? Why am I so unproductive? And undisciplined? Why? Why? Why? Sometimes his guilt would get so bad that he would start crying, wondering if he would live the rest of his life in a constant battle of wanting to do the right thing.

Salzgeber finally got to the point where enough was enough, and he said to himself, "This needs to stop. I'm am tired of this bullshit. I will figure out this procrastination thing, even if I go crazy doing it!" In the heat of that moment, he made a *commitment* to do whatever it took to stop procrastinating. And it worked. He ordered a slew of procrastination books on Amazon and started to experiment with the techniques until he found the ones that worked for him. Now a successful author himself, here's how he describes the transformation in his life.

> *I can easily get up early every morning. I take cold showers, meditate, and exercise every day. I can get things done whether I feel like it or not. I feel like I'm calling the shots. I feel powerful, and more importantly, I feel like I'm in full control of my life.*

Salzgeber says that the main technique he uses is something similar to the Peace Process, where you first become aware that you are procrastinating or you are about to procrastinate. Then,

> *You resist the urge to run away and simply stay put. You observe the negative emotions in you and experience your bodily sensations in a nonjudgmental way, without trying to change anything. You let everything just be as it is. It's all good. You're accepting that you're feeling this way right now.*

After about 30 seconds of simply observing the feeling in his body, Salzgeber starts to work on whatever task he has been avoiding. Within five minutes the negative feeling will be almost completely gone, he begins to make progress on the task, starts to feel good about himself, and becomes even more motivated to succeed.

Salzgeber's book provides a number of other techniques to help his readers overcome procrastination, but theoretically he believes that becoming aware of when you procrastinate and then focusing on the feeling in your body for a short time is all you need to stop doing it. That's exactly what I've found with the Peace Process. Only with the Peace Process, if you keep your focus on the feeling in your body for long enough to completely release it (get the intensity down to zero or one), the feeling usually won't get triggered again in the future, at least not in that situation with that particular task.

In other words, this type of mind-body technique will break the primary pattern of procrastination that happens when an uncomfortable feeling automatically makes you avoid the task you need to get done. And just like that, with something that often takes only minutes, you may have the opportunity to go from a chronic procrastinator to a successful author—or whatever you want to be.

23. Ask yourself, "What's the lesson I need to learn?"

Ask this question after you realize you have procrastinated. Another way of stating this same question is to ask, "If I had this to do over again, what would I do differently?" or "How can I make this better next time?" With this strategy, you reflect back on what happened that caused you to procrastinate on one of your goals and identify the lesson or lessons, the invaluable information you can learn from your failure or partial success that will help you be more likely to succeed in the future. This is the silver lining of your procrastination, the hidden gem of truth that we discussed when you were changing the ending to your procrastination story. Answer these questions either in your head or by writing them down.

- Think of one of the last times you procrastinated. When was it?
- What did you plan to do?
- What did you do instead?
- What triggered you? Was it a thought, an emotion, some distraction in your environment?
- If you had it to do over again, what would you do differently?
- What is the main lesson or takeaway from this experience?

When you figure out what you will do differently the next time this happens, you can also visualize yourself successfully doing that the next time you procrastinate in that situation. This will help program your mind for success and is described further in the next strategy.

24. Use visualization.

Just like when we dream at night, our minds often use pictures to communicate. The saying by Fred Bernard that "One picture is worth a thousand words" acknowledges how efficient a single picture can be. The late Steve Jobs mastered this technique as a marketing tactic when he would introduce a new Apple product by simply showing a picture of that product, using no written words. You can capitalize on this characteristic of your brain by using pictures to program your mind for whatever you might want to achieve. This strategy can be used in several different ways.

- **Visualize your intended outcome**. What will it look like when you are 100 percent successful with your goal? If you also imagine what your success will sound like and feel like, the visualization becomes even more effective. You already learned how to do this when you did the sport psychology imagery at the end of Chapter Two, when you picked a goal you wanted to achieve by the time you finished reading this book.

- **Create a vision board.** Another variation of this technique is where you find actual pictures of what you want to bring into your life in the future, paste those pictures onto what is called a **vision board**, then look at your board every day. You can use poster board, canvas, printer paper, or other materials for the board itself. Then attach pictures cut out of magazines, photos of you and others, maybe some of your favorite quotes, and anything else that inspires you. It will end up being a collage. Regularly looking at your board is another way to program your mind to move toward your goals. A lot of people swear by this technique because they manifested the goals they had pictured, sometimes in far less time than they expected.

- **Use behavior-stopping visualization.** A third way to visualize is what I call **behavior-stopping visualization**. This is where you imagine a picture in your head that would represent you, when you are doing something you *don't* want to do, like procrastinating. Think of a picture that would show you how wasteful or futile your efforts are, and how your procrastination is just a stall tactic that doesn't take you any closer to your goals. The pictures that people come up with are usually unique but meaningful to them.

I have several pictures that demonstrate this technique. One is where I am driving my car in circles around a cul-de-sac, going nowhere. I can turn my car in circles to the left or I can turn my car in circles to the right, but either way I don't make any progress. Once I learned this technique, I used it to cut back on the time I spent scrolling online news sites. As I was scrolling, I could "see" this picture in my head and I could more quickly stop and get back to doing something productive.

This type of visualization can help you break bad habits as fast or faster than many other techniques because it creates an aversion from wanting to do them in the first place. That means it can work before you procrastinate and during the time you are procrastinating. So right now, think of a picture that symbolizes you when you are procrastinating. Imagine it in detail in your mind. You can also write it down in your journal or wherever you are keeping other writing you're doing with this book. Then remember your picture the next time you catch yourself doing one of your avoidance activities. Keep practicing this visualization until the picture automatically pops up in your brain each time you fall into one of your unnecessary delays.

If you're more of an auditory person than a visual person, you can modify this technique by thinking of a phrase or sentence to say either out loud or just silently in your head when you find yourself procrastinating. For example, if you realize you are scrolling through Facebook when you need to be working on a goal, you can say to yourself something like, "What am I doing? This has nothing to do with my goal." Or maybe, "Here I am, wasting time again." Find a phrase or sentence that works for you. Again, nothing too harsh or critical.

• **Anticipate regret.** You can also use visualization and imagery to help make decisions. Let's say you need to make a decision right now. Project yourself five years into the future and imagine you have made a decision to do or not do something. You are looking back on what has happened in the past five years as a result of which decision you made. You can clearly see the consequences of your choice.

Then ask yourself, "Would I regret this?" Don't overthink your answer. Listen to your gut reaction, whatever first pops into your head. Most people get an immediate "Yes" or "No" answer. If your first attempt at this strategy doesn't tell you exactly what decision to make, keep practicing until your anticipation of regret becomes a trustworthy barometer of which way to go when you have a choice to make.

This was one of the main techniques I used when I was writing my first book. When I hit those inevitable walls and wanted to quit, I would imagine that I was at the end of my life, looking back on my decision. Would I regret it if I didn't finish my book? The answer was always a resounding "Yes!" I knew I didn't want to live (or die) with that regret, so I would dig even deeper inside of myself and find a way to keep writing.

25. Act "as if."

Do you remember playing "Pretend" when you were a child? Many children naturally take on different roles during their play, pretending to be someone they would like to become. One of the reasons this strategy can be so effective is because it puts you into the mental and emotional state of your desired future before it happens. Plus, by pretending to do something you may be afraid to do, you can sometimes learn firsthand that moving out of your comfort zone isn't going to put you in danger after all. Pretending can also be effective if you experience **imposter syndrome**, where even trying to be successful in certain areas makes you feel like a fraud or like you don't deserve it.

This strategy is similar to **role playing**, where you practice doing what you want to do. Most of my clients notice changes in their bodies right away when they role play being successful in different situations. Usually, their posture improves and they stand up taller, their breathing becomes deeper and slower, they walk with a firmer, longer stride, and their voice sounds more confident. Their thinking also changes. They become not just optimistic, but almost certain in that moment that their success is already real. Just as we can choose whatever thoughts we want, our brains have the ability to take on any role we choose. My observations with my clients are further validation that strategies like the power pose and "Fake it until you make it" actually work.

For a few minutes each day, pretend you have already reached your goals. It might be a word, a sentence, or some behavior, even if done when you're all alone. Look in the mirror and say, "Way to go!" Let yourself breathe deeper as you think *I made it!* Keep a greeting card on your desk that says "Congratulations!" Pretend with the mindset that your procrastination days are in the past and you are already a stunning success. What would that look like? How would that feel? Play. Have fun with it. Let your imagination help make your goals a reality.

26. Feel gratitude NOW.

As many people have found, gratitude is a superpower that is easily accessible and free for the taking. You can use your thoughts, your self-talk, and the images in your head to create a feeling of gratitude. That grateful feeling can override negative emotions and change your mindset—instantly. For instance, it's difficult to feel fear and gratitude at the same time, so if you're scared and want to get past that, think of something you're thankful for and let the gratitude help diminish your fear. You can even say something to yourself like, "I'm so grateful for _____ in my life." Fill in the blank. In general, gratitude can be used in three ways.

- **Feel grateful for things that are already in your life.** The list of things to feel grateful for in your life right now is endless. It includes the roof over your head, the people, the money that supports you, your health. Even the eyesight you have to be reading this book is a blessing and a gift. To feel grateful now, simply think of these blessings one by one and think of how thankful you are for them. You can also see an image in your head or look at an actual picture of one of your blessings, like a loved one, then remind yourself of how thankful you are for that person. You may find it more helpful to make a list of your blessings or simply say out loud, "I am so grateful for _____."

  Some people like to use a journal and write down at least three things they are grateful for every day. This simple practice causes you to focus on what you have instead of focusing on what you don't have. If you do this regularly, it can help you develop an abundance mindset about your life instead of a scarcity mindset. As author Eckhart Tolle says, "Acknowledging the good that you already have in your life is the foundation for all abundance." Willie Nelson said it like this, "When I started counting my blessings, my whole life turned around."

- **Feel grateful for things you want to have in your life in the future but are not yours—yet.** Gratitude before the fact is a powerful way to set the stage for your goals to manifest. Here, you can visualize your future success and what it will look like when your reach your goals. The images in your head will usually cause you to feel happy and grateful that you are already successful. You can also use actual pictures of your future success to tap into this feeling, like with a vision board. Or like how I put a picture of the front cover of this book on my refrigerator as I was writing it.

- **Feel grateful for the activities you procrastinate on.** This technique is similar to what we covered earlier, where you felt grateful for the lessons you learned from your procrastination story. Only here, gratitude can help you get through your resistance to doing a task in the moment, as you are doing it. Sometimes this only requires a simple shift in the way you think about a task you want to avoid. For example, if you don't like to exercise, rather than telling yourself, "I *have* to work out," instead say, "I *get* to work out." This shift in perspective can help you remember all the blessings that make it possible for you to exercise, like the time to work out, a place to exercise, and the physical abilities you have to do your workout.

A friend of mine, Paige, told me she doesn't like to unload the dishwasher, so she tends to procrastinate on getting it done. Paige learned that if she shifted her focus to all the reasons she was thankful for the opportunity to unload the dishwasher, it immediately helped her get past her resistance. She would say things to herself like, "I'm so grateful I have a dishwasher, that I have clean water to use, that I can afford to pay my water bills, and that I am physically capable of unloading the dishes." The gratitude she felt by shifting her focus helped her put the dishes away right then. It was that easy.

I encourage you to experiment with at least one of these types of gratitude. To get started, just for three days in a row, say or write down at least one thing you're thankful for and see what happens. After those three days, you may want to continue even longer. If you keep going, who knows? You could end up being like Willie Nelson and have your whole life turn around.

27. Feed your mind with positive influences.

I encourage you to do this last strategy at every stage of the procrastination cycle—before, during, and after. It's based on the fact that our brains are hardwired to notice negative, shocking, and potentially dangerous events in our environment far more than they notice positive events. Some say we are six time more likely to notice the negative over the positive, which makes perfect sense from a physical safety and survival standpoint.

A number of years ago, the news media discovered that negative news gets more attention from people than positive news. Since then, there has been an increasing focus on the negative, and news headlines are often written to trigger our fear. More attention from viewers and listeners, and more online views and "clicks" mean better ratings, more advertising, and more money in the pockets of producers. But the media isn't solely to blame. We are also involved. They give us more of what we say we want by what we click on.

Whether you know it or not, those frightening news stories trigger your limbic system's fight, flight, or freeze response and create an underlying, ongoing stress response within your body. Not to mention how that exposure to negativity causes you to develop more of a fixed, fearful, and helpless mindset in general. It drains your physical, mental, and emotional energy.

Each of us needs to take responsibility to limit our exposure to the news and other sources of negativity. Nurturing a growth mindset based on hope, optimism, and a can-do attitude will work wonders to help propel you toward success, especially when you are trying to achieve your more challenging goals. That means we need to not only reduce the amount of negativity in our lives, we also need to flood our minds with positive, uplifting and inspiring influences. **Overall, you want to create an 80/20 balance—80 percent positive influences and no more than 20 percent negative influences.**

Here are some suggestions. Keep your exposure to the news down to twenty minutes a day. That's usually enough time for most people to know what's going on and how to take care of themselves. You may even want to periodically take a news break and stop watching the news altogether. Don't get sucked into the fear, anger, and complaints from online feeds. Also limit your contact with negative and pessimistic people. Eliminate as many sources of negativity as you can. Instead do things like: fill your head with positive affirmations, read uplifting material, watch inspirational movies, listen to affirming and encouraging music, and surround yourself with optimistic, growth-minded people. We tend to take on the habits and characteristics of the people we spend the most time with. I suggest you find ways to spend time with people who are ahead of you in the areas where you want to grow, even if it's through reading their books or through online connections where you can benefit from their advice and from the lessons they have already learned.

I used to watch much more news than I do now. And of course, the majority of that news was negative and scary. Sometimes I would wake up in the night and be vaguely aware of thoughts about something frightening I'd seen on the news, and I would realize I was worrying about it in my sleep. Now that I've cut back on my exposure to news, I feel less anxious and more optimistic and hopeful. This change is also related to all the positive influences I experience during the day, including the upbeat, positive music I listen to, especially when I'm in my car. Now, sometimes I wake up in the night and will "hear" a line to one of the songs I've been listening to playing in my head. It makes for a much better night's sleep. Plus, I wake up in a great mood and ready to enjoy the day.

That's it. Over twenty techniques that can change your life. As I mentioned earlier, I suggest you do the first eight activities in order, then experiment with the others over time, giving each a fair trial until you find the ones that work best for you. That may mean coming back to this chapter again and again. But for right now, pat yourself on the back for at least reading through the tips and tools that can help you step into your power and your potential.

When I look back on all the years I procrastinated, it seems I was like a dog chasing its own tail. Turning in circles faster and faster, trying harder and harder in my efforts to finally achieve the success I wanted but never quite getting there. That's because just like driving around a cul-de-sac, chasing my tail was never going to get me where I wanted to go. I needed an entirely different approach to reaching my goals. That's what I mean when I say that the way or ways you have been trying to overcome your procrastination may have been part of the problem. You have just been given a new set of strategies to use, ones which address the underlying reasons you have struggled with procrastination in the first place.

At first, you may only be able to see your procrastination after the fact. However, as your awareness increases, you will get better at recognizing when you are procrastinating, during the time you are doing it. And finally, you will be able to anticipate the situations where you will be vulnerable to getting off track and stop that from happening—before you fall into your avoidance patterns. As William Blake so aptly put it

Hindsight is a wonderful thing, but foresight is better.

Overall, the goal is prevention. As you continue to use these techniques, you can start to prevent your procrastination more often. Focusing on your goals becomes enjoyable when you can see in advance where you might get stuck, then bypass the problem in advance and just keep marching forward. You get a double dose of dopamine when you become highly accomplished with your procrastination skills, *and* you fly through your to-do lists like there's no tomorrow. Plus, you don't need tomorrow to get so many things done. You're already doing more of them today.

There's even more exciting news ahead. After you bypass or remove your internal obstacles (the 80 percent of what's holding you back), you will likely find that the standard Outer Game suggestions for procrastination, goal setting, time management, and creating new habits will finally work for you. Even if they don't work right away, you will know how to use the Inner Game strategies described in this chapter to release any remaining internal resistance until you reach a point where you can benefit from Outer Game strategies. The next chapters include both Inner Game and Outer Game tips, tools, and techniques to help you succeed. Get ready to pick up speed.

Chapter 5 Highlights

Way to go! You made it to the end of the fifth chapter. You're on a roll now. Hang in there and keep going. More momentum, speed, and success are just around the corner. Here are some of the important highlights to take from this chapter.

1. Well-known procrastinators include talented people like architect Frank Loyd Wright, painter Leonardo da Vinci, and musical virtuoso Wolfgang Amadeus Mozart. These procrastinators have taught us that clearly, overcoming procrastination is not a matter of intelligence. Even geniuses have had their share of struggles.

2. As procrastinators, we are fortunate to be living now, when information recently discovered through neuroscience, coaching, and psychology allows us to work *with* our conscious and subconscious minds to overcome our unnecessary delays.

3. This chapter describes more than twenty Inner Game techniques to help you stay on track or get back on track—for use before, during and after you procrastinate. For example, let go of overcommitments, identify your procrastination triggers, make a win-win agreement between your Inner Child and you Inner Adult, and use the four-step Peace Process.

4. At first, you may only be able to see your procrastination after the fact. But as you increase your awareness, you will begin to catch your procrastination when it is happening. And finally, you will learn how to anticipate when you might procrastinate in the future and

plan ways to avoid falling into that hole. The overall goal here is prevention.

5. When you start to learn new strategies and master new skills, you will finally be able to achieve your goals. You will also be rewarded with lots of dopamine, which makes you feel energized, excited, and happy to keep going.

6. Once you learn techniques to get past the Inner Game obstacles, the ones in your mind, you will likely find that the standard Outer Game advice on topics like on time management and goal setting will also be helpful.

Action Steps

When it comes to overcoming procrastination, no one size fits all. Each of us is unique and we all learn in different ways. That means you need to use a detective mindset to solve the mystery of which strategies will help you achieve your goals. Test them and let the results speak for themselves. Sometimes finding one or two techniques is all you need to stop procrastinating and start becoming more productive.

1. Experiment with the techniques you think might be effective for you and give each one a fair trial. Read through the descriptions of the strategies and see if you can get an intuitive sense of which ones to test first.

2. Write down the techniques you test and the results you get. Use the results to identify which techniques are a good fit for you.

3. Keep coming back to this chapter, especially when you get stuck. Review what has worked for you in the past and try one or more additional strategies that might lead you to success. Keep adding to your list of strategies that work.

4. Your goal is to eventually fill your toolbox with tips and techniques that work in different situations so you never have to stay stuck in your delays, at least not for long. At that point, you're ready to spread your wings and start to fly.

Chapter 6

Goal Setting that Accelerates Your Success

As I walked through the store, my eyes latched onto a small item that I liked immediately. So I bought it. Shortly after that, I realized the item would make a great stocking gift, and I went back and bought five more. That was in July. I can't tell you how overjoyed I felt, knowing I had already done part of my Christmas shopping—six months ahead of time. I had never done that before, and I even wrote an article about it called "Christmas Shopping in July." As a recovering procrastinator, every "first" has been a cause for celebration, every milestone in my success a reason to pump my fists.

Setting early deadlines is one of the strategies we will cover in this chapter, along with celebrating milestones and successes. These strategies will help you feel empowered and give you more motivation to keep going. They give you a shot of dopamine that tells your brain, "That feels good. Do it again!" Goal setting becomes a whole new experience when you use strategies that set you up for success. As a procrastinator, changing the *ways* you go about setting and focusing on your goals can make all the difference in whether you reach them.

Many excellent books on goals are available, and much of the online advice for achieving your goals can be helpful. The vast majority of that material describes Outer Game techniques for changing your behavior and *doing* things differently. Now that you know how to move past your impulsiveness and the internal blocks that your limiting beliefs create, this material can provide a wealth of tips and tools for reaching your goals. After reading many of these books, I selected the information in this chapter based on the Outer Game and Inner Game techniques I have found to be the most effective, both from personal experience and from many years of helping my students and coaching clients achieve what they want.

What Goals Do You Want to Achieve?

When I ask people in my classes and workshops to set goals, I'm always amazed at how quickly and easily they come up with ten to twelve goals without much thought. It's as if our goals live inside of us, just waiting for the opportunity to be acknowledged and brought to life. Now is the time for you to give your goals a chance to be recognized so they can start to become part of your reality. Let's start with your BIG goals and then zero in on smaller goals you want to accomplish more immediately.

In his book, *Five Wishes*, psychologist Gay Hendricks tells this story. One time he reluctantly went to a party, mostly out of obligation to the party host, and not expecting to connect with many of the people who were there. About an hour after he got to the party, he started talking with a gentleman who looked as uncomfortable about being there as he was. As it turned out, this man was a famous spiritual teacher. Their conversation quickly went to a deeper level, and at one point, the gentleman rather abruptly suggested that Hendricks imagine he was on his deathbed and someone asked him if his life was a success. When Hendricks said "No," the man asked him to identify five things he would need to accomplish in order for his life to be successful. I'm paraphrasing, but this was the question:

What five things would you need to accomplish in order to feel successful at the end of your life?

Answering that question changed Hendrick's life. Your answers may help steer you in a direction that will change the course of your life as well. The fact that the book became a New York Times bestseller suggests that it has already helped thousands of others clarify what is most important to them.

Right now, go back to where you are keeping the writing you do with this book. Just off the top of your head, without overthinking your answers, write down five things you would need to achieve by the end of your lifetime in order to feel successful. This will only take a few minutes.

Answering this question can help you identify big-picture goals, ones that are important to you, perhaps without yet realizing they are important. Plus, your responses usually reflect your values and may help clarify your purpose in life. You may not want to work directly on any of your big, end-of-life goals now, but they give you a destination, a place where you want to end up. This means you are following this next advice on goal setting that is so often helpful:

Begin with the end in mind.

Figuring out where you want to end up at your final destination allows you to then work backwards on how you are going to get there. It's like reverse engineering your goals.

For right now, though, put your end-of-life goals aside. You identified them and got them down in writing. Even if you don't remember each one exactly the way you wrote it, trust that they are now stored in your memory somewhere in the back of your mind. Because these goals usually show us our values, priorities and life purpose, they can form a foundation for smaller goals you may want to achieve, whether or not you are consciously aware of their influence.

Make a Top Ten Goals List

A second step in our goal setting process is to identify the goals you want to accomplish at this point in your life. Our goals often change over time. What was important to achieve at age twenty may be completely different than what you want to achieve when you're forty. By the same token, some goals remain the same throughout our lives, including the big-picture, end-of-life goals you wrote down earlier.

When I ask clients to pick a goal to work on, they usually say they want to achieve a certain outcome, like making a certain amount of money. They want to *start* doing things that will help them attain their goal. Others want to *stop* doing something, like criticizing their spouse or eating so much junk food. Either way, whether you want to start or stop a behavior, it's important to get clear about where that behavior will lead and the end result you want to achieve.

Take the next five minutes or so, and just off the top of your head, without overthinking your answers, write down at least ten goals you want to accomplish. These may be big, long-term goals, or they may be smaller, more short-terms goals. They may also be steps toward accomplishing your long-term goals, but they are things you either need or want to focus on now.

After you have made your list, take another few minutes to look it over and see if there's anything you want to add or change. When you identified your problem procrastination activities earlier, there may have been some tasks that needed your more immediate attention to prevent negative consequences in the future. If you haven't already included them, add those to your top ten list. Keep this list with the other writing you are doing for this book. And put a date on it.

The rest of this book will give you lots of ways to practice achieving your goals. I suggest that you pick one of the goals from your Top Ten Goals list, something you want to achieve in the next few weeks, and use it as your **practice goal** as you go through the rest of the chapters. You may want to select more than one, depending on how many steps are involved in achieving those in the next several weeks. Unless you have already achieved the goal you set in Chapter Two—the one you want to achieve by the time you finish reading this book—you may want to use that as your practice goal.

When you achieve your practice goal (or goals), it will provide concrete evidence that you can be successful at overcoming your procrastination. You will end up feeling stronger, happier and more confident, knowing you have developed the skills to be successful. You will get that double dose of dopamine. One dose for achieving the specific goal you selected, and the other dose from learning the new skills you needed to stop procrastinating. At that point, dopamine will start to flow when you even *think* about achieving more goals and becoming more productive, and it will tell your brain, "I love this feeling. I want to do this again." What a fun way to start getting things done.

Create A Success Plan

The success rates for New Year's resolutions are abysmal. Research shows that around 80 percent of people give up on their goals by the second week in February. The majority of them quit even sooner—by January 19th to be exact. Why do so many people give up so quickly? I think the main reason is that most people never develop a plan for how they are going to achieve their goals. They head into the New Year with an *idea* for a goal—not a plan. In contrast, according to one study, people who take a few minutes to create a Success Plan are as much as twelve times more likely to be successful. Here's your chance to create a solid plan for the goal you want to achieve. All you need to do is write down your practice goal according to these guidelines.

1. **Make your goal specific and measurable.**

   Let's say your goal is to exercise more. "To exercise more" is vague, and it would be hard to measure your progress. Instead, you could describe your goal like this:

   To walk for 20 minutes three times a week.

   Do you see how much more specific that is? And how you would be able to evaluate whether or not you were successful with your goal? Okay. Write down your goal so it's specific and measurable.

2. **Make your goal realistic.**

   Setting unrealistic goals is probably the most common mistake I see people make when deciding what goals to set. For example, several of my clients set a goal to "Work out at the gym for one hour five days a week." When I asked them how many times they were currently going to the gym they said, "None." Or "Once."

   Most of us can't dramatically change our behavior overnight. It usually takes some time to start doing something consistently. A more realistic goal for these people was

   To work out at the gym for one hour twice a week.

   Once they were consistent in going to the gym twice a week for over a month, they were able to successfully increase the number of times they went. But they did it gradually.

   Another common mistake people make is setting a goal to control something that is out of their control. For example, several of my university students set a goal to get an instructor to change their grade on an exam. But just as none of us can control how other people respond to our requests, these students couldn't control what their instructors did. So the students changed their goal to this:

   Do my best when I ask my instructor to change my grade.

   The students could control how well they prepared and how appropriately assertive they were when they asked for a grade change. Even if the instructor said "No" to their request, these students could still be 100 percent successful with their goal if they did their best when speaking with the instructor. When you write down your own goal, make sure it is realistic and something you can control.

3. Pick the right time to work on your goal.

Scheduling a good time to work on your goal makes it more likely to happen. Let's say you want to go to the gym twice a week. Maybe the best time would be right after work. If that's the case, your goal might be

Work out at the gym for one hour right after work on Mondays and Thursdays.

Then make it as easy as possible to succeed at your goal by doing things like packing your gym bag the night before with workout clothes, snacks and extra water, and taking your bag to work with you in the morning so you can drive straight to the gym.

Another aspect of picking the right time is to work on your goal when you have the time and energy to add something new to your life. If you already feel stressed and overwhelmed by the responsibilities you currently have in your life, you may need to either cut back on your other obligations or decide to wait for a better time to work on your goal. My sense is that working on New Year's resolutions at the first of the year isn't great timing for many people.

4. Set a deadline.

Some goals have definite endpoints when they get completed, and some goals are more like ongoing habits (like walking twice a week). Goals that don't have an endpoint tend to lose their urgency and drag on and on if they lack a deadline. Deadlines give us a time frame for completing our goals, a date to work toward. That means we are more likely to be motivated to continue working on our goals until we get to the finish line. I'm now working on a deadline to finish this book, which is to

Complete my book by August 16, 2023 by writing three hours during the Golden Hours, five days a week.

According to recent research, defining your deadline by smaller units of time instead of some vague time in the future makes it more likely you will succeed. For example, I can feel my energy increase when I say my goal is to

Complete my book in the next 87 days by writing three hours during the Golden Hours, five days a week.

A deadline described by the remaining days available brings a different level of reality to the time you have left and often increases your energy and sense of urgency around your goal (and sometimes a healthy amount of anxiety). I encourage you to give your goal a deadline that you describe in days, hours or even minutes, depending on the kind of goal it is. Also, be sure your deadlines are realistic. Remember, procrastinators tend to overestimate the amount of time they have to complete a goal and underestimate the amount of time it will take to complete it.

5. **Identify your WHY.**

Writing down a Success Plan for each of your goals increases your chances of success, as does identifying your WHY and writing that down. WHY do you want to achieve your goal? What is your motivation? Look deep inside yourself and figure out why your goal is important to you.

For instance, you might want to lose weight so you will look good at your high school reunion. But what happens when your reunion is over? What will motivate you to keep the weight off? Motivation that is based on pleasing or impressing others is often not as strong as being motivated by deeply personal reasons that relate to your values. For example, if you want to lose weight so you will be healthy enough to be a good parent for your children, that WHY can help you stay motivated to maintain your weight loss long into the future. You can have more than one WHY for each of your goals. Look for at least one WHY for your practice goal that is tied to your values and write that down.

I can't over-emphasize the importance of taking just a few minutes to create your Success Plan by following these five guidelines. According to a study done by Gail Matthews at Dominion University, **you are 39.5 percent more likely to complete your goals—just by writing them down.** Getting your goals *and* your Success Plan down in writing will definitely help tip the odds of success in your favor.

Here's How to Make Your Success Plan Even Better

The steps in the Success Plan I just described are standard advice from experts in the fields of self-improvement, goal setting, time management, and productivity. These steps are often referred to as setting **SMART goals**, which is an acronym for Specific, Measurable, Achievable, Realistic, and Timely. I worded them a little differently and included a few extra suggestions, but they're basically the same. There's tons of research to show that following these steps will increase your chances of succeeding at your goals, especially if you visualize the outcomes you want, like with the sport psychology imagery described at the end of Chapter Two.

Many people find that by following these steps, they get what they want—and then some. That's why I suggest you write down and visualize your goals, but also allow for the possibility that you may achieve something even greater. In fact, it's a good idea to add to the end of every goal statement a phrase that says, **"This or something better."**

If you have a more vague or general goal, like to be happy, or if you don't know exactly *how* to achieve your goal—what specific steps to take—don't give up. Do whatever seems like it might move you toward the outcome you want. *And* be open to unusual and unexpected events in your life that could help you get there. In other words, know what you want, even if it's just a general idea. Take action on that idea, but don't get too focused on exactly *how* you will achieve it. Be open to the unexpected, like epiphanies, coincidences and so-called "accidents." And allow for the possibility that when you reach your goals, your results will be much better than you could have ever imagined.

Plan for Your Success—and Plan for Your Failure

Whether you know exactly what goals you want and how to achieve them, or whether your goals are more like vague desires, the journey toward completing your goals is rarely a straight line. You will zig zag. Run into roadblocks. Slide off to the side of the road. You may get frustrated and impatient with how long it's taking you to get where you want to go. You may fall back into old ways of thinking that undermine your self-confidence and motivation. Some days may feel easy and you can succeed almost without trying. Other days, you may get so discouraged that you want to give up. At times, you may feel like you're a complete failure. All of that—and more— can happen to squelch your efforts. Even the best-laid Success Plans can, and often do, run amuck. Consider this quote by Winston Churchill.

The definition of success is going from failure to failure without losing your enthusiasm.

None of us likes to fail. But failure is part of the road to success. And it gets easier once you accept the fact that sometimes you're going to mess up, you're going to make mistakes, and you're going to do things wrong. **The paradox of success is that the more you embrace failure and learn from it, the more likely you are to succeed**. The point is to know that in advance and to have a plan for how you are going to keep the inevitable setbacks, failures and disasters from blocking your progress.

Kelly McGonigal is a health psychologist who teaches a course on willpower through the Stanford University School of Medicine. In her class, students set a willpower goal at the beginning of the semester to either start doing something (train for a marathon, become a better parent) or stop doing something (quit smoking, resist chocolate). The class is open to the public, and it became so popular that she had to keep finding a larger room to accommodate all the students. Through teaching this class multiple times, McGonigal learned some key lessons from her students, which she writes about in her book *The Willpower Instinct*. She states, "I believe that the best way to improve your self-control is to see how and why you lose control. Knowing how you are likely to give in doesn't, as many people fear, set yourself up for failure. It allows you to support yourself and avoid the traps that lead to willpower failures." According to McGonigal, **the main reason people lose control and fail at their goals is because, "They fail to predict when, where, and why they will give in."**

Here's your chance to set yourself up for success with your own goals. Look back at your track record of achieving goals in your life. What obstacles did you run into that caused you to fail at your goals? Was it something in your environment, an Outer Game obstacle, that stopped your progress toward your goal, like not enough time? Also, what patterns do you see in yourself—your Inner Game obstacles—that tend to block your success? Do you overcommit and then feel overwhelmed? Do you get bored with your goals or lose interest and then give up? Do you impulsively default to your favorite avoidance activities (like going online) when your goals get hard? Be honest with yourself and identify what it is about you that could cause you to give up.

Think about your practice goal, then start to create your Plan for Failure by writing down your answers to these next three questions. If you're working on an easy goal, your answers may be short. For harder goals, you may have a longer list of possible obstacles.

1. **WHEN will I be most likely to give up on my goal?**
   Will it be when something happens in my environment, like I get sick or bad weather makes it too hard to exercise outdoors? And what do I know about myself, my Inner Game patterns, that could get in the way of my success? Will I get too discouraged to keep going when more obstacles show up than I expected? Write down your own answers.

2. **WHERE am I likely to give in and abandon my goal?**
   Will it be when I'm traveling away from home and don't have my normal daily routine to help make sure I exercise in the morning? Will I be more likely to cave into the temptation to eat sugar when I'm at work? Write down where you might be the most vulnerable.

3. **WHY will I fail at achieving my goal?**
   What Outer Game and Inner Game obstacles could cause me to fail? And why would those obstacles make me give up? Will it be because of something in my environment, like I don't have enough support from other people? Could it be because of something within myself, like I misjudged how long it would take to reach a goal and started thinking it wasn't worth it. Again, write down your own why.

The next step in creating your Plan for Failure is to write down what you will do *instead* of giving up on your goal. In other words, how you are going to prevent those obstacles from squashing your efforts? How are you going to avoid failure and keep marching forward? Here are a few examples.

Outer Game obstacle: The schedule of classes at my gym will change so I can't go to the class I want anymore.

Plan for Success: I will find another class or another gym that accommodates my available time. Or I will find online classes so I can work out at home. Or I will make up my own workout routine and do that on my own. I'll work out to music so it will be more fun.

Inner Game obstacle: I will underestimate the time and effort it takes to complete my goal. It will take longer and be harder than I expected. This will become so discouraging that I'll want to say, "Just forget it."

Plan for Success: I will use the golden hours to whittle away at the steps required to complete my goal, no matter how long it takes. And when I get discouraged, I will remember WHY my goal is important and repeat affirmations that inspire me to keep going.

Write down your own Outer Game and Inner Game obstacles, along with your plans for success. As you work toward completing your practice goal, use your detective mindset to move past any obstacles that might get in your way. Here's a heads up. Many life coaches who work on goal setting with their clients have found that people tend to give up on their goals after anywhere from twenty-one to forty-five days, for various reasons. Your vulnerable times may be longer or shorter time periods than that, but your detective mindset will help you look for patterns in *when* you fail, as well as *where* and *why* you fail. Then learn the lessons your failures have to teach you and turn those lessons into strategies that help you succeed the next time.

Here's another heads up. Throughout your journey to overcome procrastination, it's important to have a definition of failure that can help move you forward. At an early age, most of us get taught to believe that mistakes and failures are bad, and we should avoid them at all costs. **But what we call failures are simply messages telling you to do something different**. To move in another direction. Try something else. Each mistake and failure has at least one valuable lesson embedded in it, a nugget of wisdom that can help you achieve your goals. Please don't beat yourself up when you make mistakes or interpret your "failures" as something you did wrong. **Sometimes you need to know what doesn't work in order to figure out what does**. It's all a part of learning.

Besides, people who are more compassionate and forgiving toward themselves are more likely to succeed. They don't carry the burden of guilt that can be so crippling, especially when they're focused on more challenging goals. Ask yourself, "Do I get self-critical when I fail?" If your answer is "Yes," please, cut yourself some slack. Find some positive and encouraging things you can say to yourself like, "Failures and mistakes are a normal part of learning how to do something new. I'm working on getting better at this. I'm moving in the right direction and I'm on the right track. I know I'll eventually get there. In the meantime, I deserve to feel good about my progress, so I'm going to focus on learning my lessons and enjoying the journey, failures and all." **Being kind and supporting**

yourself as you're going through this learning process will not only help you feel better, it will also help you go faster.

Experiment with These Success Strategies

After you have created your Plan for Success and your Plan for Failure, it's time to roll up your sleeves and get into the nitty-gritty of actually working on your goals. Think about what you have done in the past to reach your goals. You probably have a whole toolbox of techniques that have worked for you before. Use the strategies you're already good at. Here are a few more that my students and clients have found especially helpful.

1. **Start with easy goals.**

   By easy, I mean you are 90 to 95 percent certain you can achieve them. You can do that by either setting a small, easy goal or by focusing on a small step in reaching a bigger goal. When you succeed, your dopamine will begin to flow and your self-confidence will increase. Later on, when you become more confident with your goal-setting skills, you can set bigger and more challenging goals.

2. **Schedule time to work on your goal**.

   When you write out your Plan for Success, you will decide when you will focus on your goal. With this scheduling technique, you then break your goal into small steps and plug those steps into your calendar each day. That way you know exactly what you need to do toward achieving your goal and when you need to do it. For example, if your goal is to work out at the gym right after work on Mondays and Thursdays, schedule those times in your calendar.

3. **Overcome overwhelm.**

   When you feel overwhelmed, you may need to break your goal into even smaller steps. Then prioritize those steps and do them one at a time. Stay focused on your most important goal and save the rest of the things you need to do for later (or schedule time to do less important tasks).

4. **Do one thing toward achieving your goal.**

   When you get stuck, ask yourself, "What is one action I can take right now that will take me closer to my goal?" If you stay in motion, moving toward your goal, it will help prevent the paralysis by analysis that comes when you get caught up in your head. Another way to think of this strategy is to do the next right thing in the moment, then the next right thing, then the next.

5. **Use positive self-talk.**

When you start to get distracted from your goal, you can say things to yourself like: "Just because I want to do something else (check my phone, post to Instagram, watch Netflix) doesn't mean I have to do it. I have a CHOICE. I can work on my goal instead and end up feeling so much better about myself."

6. **Be accountable to yourself or someone else.**

Measuring your progress each day is a great way to be accountable to yourself. For example, a story is told about Jerry Seinfeld, the comedian and star of the hugely popular television sitcom "Seinfeld." When Jerry was first getting started in comedy, he set a goal to write one joke a day. He kept a month-at-a-glance calendar on his wall, and every day he wrote a joke, he would put a big red "X" on the calendar. After a while, he had a long chain of "Xs," and those motivated him to continue because he didn't want to break the chain. You can do the same thing. Find a way to keep a visual record of your success where you will see it often, and use the record of your success as motivation to keep going.

You may also want to find someone else to help provide accountability for your progress. Through her Old Dominion University research, Gail Matthews found that **people who wrote down their goals** and **were accountable to someone else were a whopping 76.7 percent more likely to achieve them**. All the participants had to do to get these stunning results was send progress reports to friends. Being accountable to a group of people can also work. Consider joining a class or group of people who can help you stay on track. Groups like WeightWatchers and Overeaters Anonymous are examples if your goal is weight loss. Many online groups of people with the same interests are available to provide the kind of support and accountability that might dramatically boost your chances of success.

Find What Works For You

Just like when you figured out which strategies help you overcome procrastination, finding goal-setting strategies that work for you comes through experimenting. Through trial and error. Through testing out different strategies and letting the results speak for themselves. That's what successful people do. They keep trying different things until they find what works.

Every year for the past twenty years, *People* magazine has published a special edition on weight loss called "Half Their Size." Their staff interviews ordinary people who have lost half their body weight through lifestyle changes, and they purposefully exclude celebrities with private chefs and personal trainers. Each special edition contains the stories of people who have been able to maintain their weight loss for at least several years.

When you read through the stories, you notice that each person found success using different techniques. Here are some examples of the lessons they learned along the way and what advice they would give to others.

- I didn't decide to lose weight until I was in my 40s. Now, 30 years later, I know you're never too old to start.
- Find out "why" you want to lose weight. Write it down and put it where you'll see it often. Every day, read it out loud.
- This isn't a race and you're not competing with anyone else. Focus on yourself and on getting better every day.
- Celebrate the small successes and the milestones. I bought new clothes for the new me as I lost the weight.
- I always show up for everyone else. Now I also show up for myself.

Your goals may not include weight loss, but the point is to find what strategies work for you regardless of your goals. There are lessons for you to learn as you start to achieve the goals that are important to you, lessons only you can discover by rolling up your sleeves, trying different techniques, and getting feedback from your efforts.

Set Goals to Stop Procrastinating

In addition to setting personal goals and using the techniques to achieve them that we have covered so far in this chapter, many people make faster progress when they also set goals to learn specific skills for overcoming procrastination. When you master a new skill that helps you stop procrastinating, it gives you that double dose of dopamine: one dose for learning something new and one dose for making progress on your original goal. Along with that dopamine usually comes a boost of energy and a burst of excitement about all the possibilities that lie ahead. Do you want to try it? Most of the following techniques will help with goal setting and with overcoming procrastination.

1. **Celebrate your successes.**

   But do this consistently, even for small achievements. Pat yourself on the back when you stay on your schedule two days in a row. Pump your fists in the air and holler "Whoo-hoo!" when you complete an important step toward one of your goals. Brag about your successes to others (just a little). Give yourself rewards for achieving goals you worked hard on. For example, at the very least, I'm giving myself a new cell phone when I finish writing this book. Rewards and celebrations help create more dopamine and happy feelings that tell your brain you have lots to look forward to when you stop procrastinating and keep plugging away at your goals. That your efforts are definitely worth it.

2. **Set early deadlines.**

   This technique was very popular with my university students. They felt relieved when they met deadlines in their classes ahead of time and didn't have to stress about their assignments at the last minute. They also felt empowered by knowing they could control their behavior well enough to put a personal deadline on a goal—before it was due—and meet it. Try turning in your taxes in March. Finish your Christmas shopping by November. Pay your bills well ahead of their due dates. Take care of a health issue before it becomes a problem. Then enjoy the good feelings that come from your early-bird efforts.

3. **Use challenges.**

   Challenges are goals you set for yourself that only last a relatively short time. Usually hours, days, weeks, or a few months. The idea behind challenges is that most of us can keep ourselves focused on achieving a goal for at least a little while. If you're successful with your challenge, you create a new normal for yourself of what you're able to do. You show yourself that you're capable of achieving more than you had in the past, so any limiting beliefs about your abilities get proven wrong. Despite some possible fears, you create proof positive that you can break through your comfort zone and not only live to tell about it, but maybe even find that life outside your old restrictions is an exhilarating place to be. Here are some suggestions.

- **Increase your phone-free time.**
  When you get up each morning, see how long you can go without checking your phone. Ten minutes? Thirty minutes? Two hours? Then see if you can increase the amount of time when you're phone free.
- **Challenge yourself to not get distracted.**
  When you're working on a goal, set a challenge to not get distracted. Each day, see how long you can work on your goal without giving in to either external distractions (the conversation in the next room) or internal distractions (frustration, your urge to go online). Time yourself and keep a record of your efforts.
- **Re-focus. Faster.**
  See how fast you can re-focus on your goal after you get distracted. Then work toward reducing the amount of time it takes to get back on task.
- **Use challenges with your most frequent blocks.**
  Identify the things that keep tripping you up as you work toward reaching your goals and set challenges for each of those. Usually these are internal blocks. For example, do you give up when you feel overwhelmed? Set a challenge to stay focused on your goal for five minutes after you notice you want to give up. Or stay focused for three minutes. Or even one minute. Stick with it for as long as you can. Let it be okay to feel overwhelmed. Then challenge yourself to stay focused for longer and longer periods of time, *while* you are feeling overwhelmed.

Challenges are sometimes referred to as "stretch goals," because you are trying to stretch yourself to reach your personal best. Your overall goal is to be better today than you were yesterday. You're not competing against anyone else. You're only competing against yourself. Against your old record. Make it a game. Play hard. Keep score. Write down how you do. Like Jerry Seinfeld, find a way to track your progress so you have visible results of your efforts.

Just make sure your challenges are realistic. They should be hard enough to make you stretch, but not so hard that you can't complete them. I suggest that you start with easy challenges so you will get the dopamine going. In the *People* magazine issue that featured sustained weight loss, one woman described how she did it like this: "I set small achievable goals. Then I worked hard to exceed them, which gave me even more motivation."

Like this woman and many of the people I have worked with, you can also set yourself up for success by choosing small achievable challenges. Do a daily review each night to help you learn your lessons and stay on track.

Every November, fiction writers can join a creative writing challenge called NaNoWriMo, which stands for National Novel Writing Month. Participants challenge themselves to write an entire novel (50,000 words) in 30 days, starting on November first. Hundreds of thousands of people from all over the world accept this challenge each year. It's like a marathon for writers. At the end of the month, writers submit their novels for judging, and prizes are given to those who meet all the requirements. This is a great example of a more difficult challenge, but one that is clearly defined and easy to measure. Challenges can go from something very small to the more extreme. You get the idea. If you decide to set challenges for yourself, be realistic about what you're capable of pulling off. However, many of us can accomplish amazing feats if we only have to do something for a short time. Plus, it can be fun to push yourself and test your abilities.

4. Break through the "Triple Whammy"

If you get stuck on a particular goal and can't seem to break through your resistance, consider using this strategy. I learned it from one of my coaches, Christian Mickelsen, who calls it the **triple whammy.** I've used it to overcome procrastination with myself, with individual clients, and with people in my groups. Just ask yourself these three questions. Thinking about the goal you're stuck on . . .

1. How do you feel about yourself, right now, knowing that you have been procrastinating on this goal? Do you feel any discomfort or angst?

2. Think about actually working on your goal to get it done. Do you feel any discomfort or angst when you think about doing whatever it will take to complete this goal?

3. Now imagine you have successfully completed your goal. Do you feel any discomfort or angst now that you have accomplished your goal?

It always surprises me how often people feel angst around all three phases of completing a goal—before, during and after. It's easy to understand feeling bad before and during the time you're working on a goal, especially if that goal is particularly difficult. But I'd say the majority of people I've asked also feel bad when they think about actually completing their goal. They usually tell me they have fears around what will happen next. Sometimes they are afraid of other people's reactions. Sometimes they have a vague fear something bad will happen if they're successful (but they're not sure what that would be). Their reasons vary, but by itself, this fear or angst can be enough to make them keep their foot on the brakes and stay stuck, even though staying stuck also makes them feel bad. Talk about a no-win situation.

So what can you do in situations like this? One technique is to identify any fears or limiting beliefs that are underneath your angst or discomfort. Then ask yourself if those fears or limiting beliefs are realistic. And even if your fears and beliefs do seem valid, ask yourself, "Is it *still* worth it to keep going, to accomplish my goal anyway, and to deal with any negative consequences later on?" Keep in mind that the consequences you imagine will happen may not happen after all. With this technique, you use logic and reasoning to work through whatever is stopping you. We covered this technique in Chapter Five (see Technique Thirteen).

Another way to break through the triple whammy is to use the Peace Process. Find the feeling of angst in your body. Keep your attention on that feeling long enough for it to get released. Do this with any uncomfortable emotion you feel when you think about the time before, during or after you achieve your goal. Once the negative feelings are released, most likely, you will be free to move forward on completing your goal.

Achieving a goal you've been stuck on for a long time can give you a thrill and a sense of accomplishment like no other. Congratulate yourself for getting unstuck, and find at least one way to celebrate your success. You also deserve a reward. After a major breakthrough, you deserve to feel rock-star phenomenal.

Troubleshooting Tips

You may have noticed a section of a product owner's manual on troubleshooting tips. It's included in most manuals, usually near the back. It gives you tips on how to get past any problems you might be having with your product working properly. That's what this section of this book is about. It gives you suggestions on what to look for if you continue to have trouble reaching your goals, despite your best efforts. Ask yourself these questions.

1. Do I have any limiting beliefs I'm not aware of that might be

holding me back?

This is one of the main reasons why people stay stuck on their goals for a long time. One way to uncover any beliefs that may be hidden is to notice what you are thinking when you try to work on your goal. Write down your thoughts, then look for any beliefs that might be underneath the thoughts.

Another way to identify any hidden beliefs is to notice how you feel when you get stuck while working on a goal. Then ask yourself, "Is this feeling familiar? Has there ever been a time in my life when I remember feeling this way when I tried to achieve a goal?" It can be especially helpful to think back to your childhood and look for any times you felt this way when you were under the age of eight. Look for any beliefs you might have learned as a child that are now holding you back. Then use the strategies in Chapter Five and other parts of this book to transform any limiting beliefs into empowering ones.

2. Am I stuck in my comfort zone?

Our subconscious mind tries to keep us safe by sounding off alarms when we try to move past our comfort zone. Your alarms may show up as fear, a racing heartbeat, procrastination, and thoughts that say "Danger ahead." This is perfectly normal and to be expected when you want to do something you've never done before. Sometimes you just need to feel the fear and do it anyway.

But what if there is real danger ahead? Sometimes our fear is trying to keep us safe. Just in case your danger signals are not false alarms, always ask yourself this question:

What's the worst that could happen?

Let's say your goal is to make more money by investing in a business opportunity. Ask yourself, "What's the worst that could happen?" If you make the investment with money you can afford to lose, then maybe there is no real danger involved. But if it's a risky deal and you can't afford to lose your investment, your subconscious may be trying to protect you from a valid and dangerous outcome. Always listen to your doubts and fears. Then evaluate the risks involved with your goals before moving forward.

Sometimes people get stuck in their comfort zone because they don't want to make other people uncomfortable. For example, I can't tell you the number of times people have told me that when they start to lose weight, others around them try to sabotage their efforts. In situations like this, **you may be moving outside someone else's comfort zone**. Often this happens because of someone else's insecurities. Maybe they don't want your relationship to change. Or maybe they feel threatened or jealous of your possible success. There can be lots of reasons why your success or potential success triggers a negative reaction in others.

Sometimes you may *anticipate* that success with your goal will make someone else uncomfortable, so you will hold back and try to prevent the other person from feeling bad. This is a classic codependent pattern, where you try to protect other people from their own feelings. It rarely works. If you hold back, you will likely end up resenting them for it, when really, you're the one who chose to abandon your goals in order to protect them. Yes, we need to be considerate and respectful of the feelings of others. But each of us needs to learn how to deal with our own emotions rather than have others try to prevent us from feeling them.

However, if you anticipate that your success will upset someone who has power over you, again ask the question, "What's the worst that can happen?" Think through the possible consequences of your success in terms of how the other person might react. Sometimes it's better to wait on your goals rather than have to deal with the other person's reaction. Anyone in an abusive relationship can probably understand the importance of waiting for the right timing. You don't want to anger a bull unless you have a way to keep yourself safe.

We bump into the edges of other people's comfort zones more often than we may realize. The key is to increase your awareness of when that happens so you can sort through your options. In many situations you can try talking with them about your concerns and see if you can work through it together. If they seem trustworthy enough, explain your goals to them and tell them how much you would appreciate their support. But make it clear that you will pursue your goals with or without their help. The bottom line is that you need people around you who will be your cheerleaders and who will support you as you move past your own comfort zone. Sometimes, the best option is to let go of the relationships that feel restrictive and bring you down (if you can), or at least minimize the amount of time you spend with those people.

Facing our fears and moving past our comfort zones can make all the difference in whether we enjoy our lives or simply endure them. Take

Carol, for example. Carol had been married for sixteen years and had four children. Sometimes she felt like her husband was another child. He only worked sporadically, leaving her to work three jobs in order to pay their bills. Their relationship eventually fell apart, and Carol made the monumental decision to get a divorce. Despite her overwhelming fear, Carol knew it was the right thing to do for her children and for herself.

I ran into Carol two years after her divorce. She said she had fallen in love with the most wonderful man and they had recently gotten engaged. He adored her children, and they already called him Dad. Carol made an interesting comment: "I was so terrified of getting a divorce. But because I did, now I'm living the life I always dreamed about." Carol had the courage to step outside her comfort zone and into the unknown. That made all the difference in creating a level of happiness in her life she had always hoped was possible.

Is it worth it to find the courage within yourself to break free from your comfort zone? If you were to ask Carol, you would get an exuberant, over-the-top, and wildly enthusiastic, "YES!"

More Troubleshooting Tips

If you don't think your limiting beliefs are holding you back, and if you're pretty sure it's not because of a fear of moving out of your comfort zone, ask yourself these additional questions.

3. Could I be depressed?
If you have felt empty, sad, hopeless or down for more than two weeks and can't get motivated, it might be depression instead of procrastination.

4. Am I overly anxious?
High anxiety levels can make it difficult to stay focused on your goals. Especially if you are overly anxious about things beyond what you procrastinate on, you may have an issue with anxiety.

5. Do I have ADHD?
Is it hard for you to concentrate on *anything* for very long, not just your more difficult goals? If so, you may have ADHD (Attention Deficit Hyperactive Disorder). This condition can cause you to be hyperactive, impulsive, and forgetful. And you may find it difficult to prioritize, avoid distractions, and stay motivated.

6. Am I sleep deprived?

Fatigue is a major reason why many people procrastinate. Not getting enough sleep can cause you to be more impulsive and distractible. Plus, you may simply not have enough energy to work on your goals.

7. Am I too stressed out?

Or am I experiencing mental or emotional burnout? Sometimes you get maxed out in terms of what you can handle. When that happens, you may need to take care of yourself before you can fully focus on your current goals or take on any new ones.

Any one of these conditions will probably need to be addressed separately. For example, if you are tired all the time, your procrastination fix may be something as simple as getting more sleep. However, if you get more sleep and you're still tired, something else might be going on. Fatigue can be a symptom of a number of health concerns. If you think any of these concerns might be holding you back—or if you suspect there might be any other issues going on with you—please see a physician or mental health professional and check for any physical or psychological reasons for your procrastination. If there are any underlying issues, then get the help you need so you can move on with your life.

8. Am I on any medications that might be contributing to my procrastination?

I also want to mention that sometimes certain medications can make it harder to get things done. For example, people who are on antidepressants or antianxiety medications often feel numb and can't feel their feelings. These medications can cause you to lose access to feelings such as hope, excitement and determination that are so important for achieving more challenging goals. That's because **to the extent that you numb any one emotion, you numb them all.** For example, to the extent you numb your sadness, you also numb your excitement. The same thing can happen with pain medications, both prescription medications and those bought over the counter.

Our feelings provide a source of energy and an emotional compass to help guide us through life. That means that people who are on certain medications may find it difficult to get better, even if they're in individual therapy. Self-help healing techniques like the Peace Process may not work because their emotional awareness is muffled. If possible, it's ideal to avoid any circumstances that cause you to lose touch with your feelings.

However, if you want to move toward getting off of any medications, always check with your doctor first and follow medical advice.

What About Addictions?

Ask yourself this additional troubleshooting question, **"Am I addicted to something?"** It is surprisingly easy to get addicted to substances (like alcohol and nicotine) as well as to certain activities or behaviors (like gambling and shopping). Addictions can severely limit your ability to live life on your own terms. When those addictions become severe, they can bring your life to a painful standstill.

More and more, we're seeing worldwide that addictions to our screens are causing a massive and exploding increase in procrastination. People are addicted to their smartphones, tablets, computers and other digital devices because those devices give them access to the internet. The internet provides instant, 24/7 access to a growing number of platforms that can become addictive, like social media and online gaming. Millions and millions of people around the world are losing control over how much time they spend looking at their screens, which means they ignore or put off doing things they either need or want to get done.

This happened to me! I got addicted to screen time when I was writing this book. In Chapter Eight, I describe more about my own internet addiction and provide suggestions on how to find a healthy balance between the real world and the online world.

What Are You Waiting For?

Before we end this chapter, ask yourself this final question, **"What could I be waiting for?"** Sometimes our procrastination throws us into a perpetual waiting game, acting as if something else needs to happen before we can start doing what we want to do. Do you know what you might be waiting to have happen before you can move forward? Maybe . . .

- You're waiting until you're not so busy.
- You're waiting until you have more money.
- You're waiting until you feel "ready" or until you feel like getting it done. (FYI, you may never feel ready and you may never feel like doing something.)
- You're waiting until you can do it "right." (You may be afraid to do something wrong so you don't do anything at all.)

- You're waiting for your fear to go away. (Hint: that may never happen. Feel the fear and do it anyway. Or deal with the danger if it's a real possibility.)
- You're waiting for someone else to give you permission. If that is what's going on with you, I am giving you permission. Here. Now. Better yet, also give *yourself* permission to move forward with your goals.
- You're waiting to stop doing things that might have worked for you in the past, but clearly don't work now. You may be afraid of feeling like a quitter. But sometimes what you're doing now is never going to work, so you need to cut your losses, learn your lessons, and do something different.

If any of these ring true for you or if other reasons to wait pop into your mind, question them. They may be valid concerns. If that's the case, then address the concern and either remove it as an obstacle or find a way around it. Because like Carol, in the long run, you will probably find that living the life of your dreams is so rich and so rewarding that it's worth every minute and every ounce of energy it takes to get there.

Now that you know how to set yourself up for success with your goals, it's time to turn your goal-setting skills into habits. Many experts agree that having clear, achievable goals for where you want to go is a necessary ingredient for a successful future. They also agree that daily habits—what you do day in and day out—are among the most important things you can do to create the life you want. Keep reading. The next chapter will tell you exactly how to break bad habits and build the good habits that can help make your dreams come true.

Also, congratulations for getting this far. You've got this. I'm cheering you on every step of the way.

Chapter 6 Highlights

According to a well-known adage: "If you don't know where you're going, you'll probably end up somewhere else." Goals are your destination, where you want your journey to take you. Goal-setting techniques include the map of how you're going to get there. Here are some highlights from this chapter.

1. As a procrastinator, changing the *ways* you go about setting and focusing on your goals can make all the difference in whether you reach them. By

using research-based techniques that help you succeed, goal setting can become a whole lot more fun.

2. You are 39.5 percent more likely to achieve your goals if you write them down. Wow.

3. The paradox of failure is that the more you embrace failure and learn from it, the more likely you are to succeed.

4. Having a Success Plan—and a Plan for Failure—increases your chances of completing your goals. Research shows that the main reason people fail at their goals is because they don't create a plan for when, where, and why they will give up.

5. One study found that people who wrote down their goals *and* were accountable to someone else for their progress were a stunning 76.7 percent more likely to achieve them. Wow again.

6. Setting specific goals to stop procrastinating gives you a double dose of dopamine: one dose for learning new skills and one dose for making progress on your original goals.

7. Now that you know how to move past your impulsiveness, comfort zone, and limiting beliefs, you will probably find that the books and online material that describe Outer Game techniques for goal setting will be immensely helpful. See the Recommended Reading section at the back of this book for suggestions.

Action Steps

This chapter covers strategies to help you win the Outer Game and the Inner Game in order to succeed at your goals. I describe the strategies below in more detail in this chapter. They don't take that long to complete. If you want to add some rocket fuel to your efforts to reach your goals, I encourage you to do them all.

1. Write down your long-term, lifetime goals by answering this question: What five things would you need to accomplish in order to feel successful at the end of your life?

2. Write down at least ten more short-term goals that you want to achieve right now.

3. Select a "practice goal" to work on as you go through the rest of this book. Write out a Success Plan and a Plan for Failure for your practice

goal according to the guidelines in this chapter.

4. Many people make faster progress when they also set goals to learn new skills for overcoming procrastination. For example, set a goal to not get distracted. Or set a goal to reduce the amount of time you spend on your phone.

5. Read through the section on Troubleshooting Tips. When you get stuck on a goal in spite of your best efforts, there may be physical or psychological issues going on. Maybe you just need more sleep. Or maybe you're depressed or overly anxious. If you think there might be underlying issues, see a physician or mental health professional so you can get unstuck and move on with your life.

Chapter 7

The Advantages of Healthy Habits

At just twenty years old, Hal Elrod had found an extraordinary level of success. He was in love with his girlfriend, was surrounded by supportive family and friends, and as a top-earning sales representative for a marketing company, he was making more money than he ever imagined.

But all of that changed in an instant. One night while driving down the freeway at seventy miles an hour, Elrod smashed head-on into a Chevy pickup that was barreling straight toward him going eighty. He doesn't remember seeing the headlights of the drunk driver who was going the wrong way, but the crash was so horrific that technically, it killed him. His heart stopped beating and he quit breathing for six minutes. Emergency rescue crews airlifted him to a hospital where he spent the next six days in a coma. When he woke up, Elrod was told he had permanent brain damage and eleven fractured bones. Doctors said he might never walk again. And his then-girlfriend broke up with him (while he was in the hospital) and suddenly became his ex.

When people go through this kind of unimaginable tragedy, they often fall into a deep depression that can be incredibly difficult to get out of. But not Elrod. He asked, "Why me?" but didn't linger on that question. He didn't feel sorry for himself. And he didn't dwell on what he couldn't change. Instead of thinking about what he didn't have, he chose to be grateful for all the things he did have. He also chose to put 100 percent of his focus on fulfilling his potential and achieving his dreams. In other words, he used positive thinking and a success mindset to catapult himself through the healing process and back into a lifestyle of abundance. It took a number of years, but he hung in there and eventually he was topping his previously best sales records. He had a thriving life coaching business, he was in demand as a motivational speaker, and he met a woman who eventually became "the one."

Elrod's success—both before and after his accident—was driven by his empowering beliefs about himself and about life. Those beliefs helped him form the day-to-day habits that allowed him to keep reaching his personal best. Probably without knowing it, Elrod also found ways to work with the psychological principles that govern habits, which meant he could break any bad habits that didn't fuel his success and build the kinds of new habits that would help him get the results he wanted. You can learn how to do the same.

How Do Habits Work?

Habits are behaviors or routines that we perform regularly. Healthy habits form the foundation of a successful life, so it's worth spending a little time to understand how they work. Consider this quote by Frank Outlaw.

Watch your thoughts, they become words;

Watch your words, they become actions;

Watch your actions, they become habits;

Watch your habits, they become character;

Watch your character, for it becomes your destiny.

Our habits start with our thoughts and our words, perhaps especially the words we say to ourselves (our self-talk). These thoughts and words become the actions and then the habits that form our character. Our character makes up much of our identity, of what kind of person we are. In large part, our identity determines our destiny. Elrod's destiny of success clearly started with his thoughts. Before his accident happened, based on his beliefs, he was in the habit of thinking positively. Despite the injuries that were caused by his crash, afterward he still thought of himself as a successful person.

All too often, however, people struggle to develop healthy habits, even when they have an identity of success and even when they practice positive thinking. Breaking bad habits and building good habits can be much easier once you understand the psychology of how habits are formed and how they are broken. There is a straightforward formula, based on psychological principles, that determines your habits. Here's the simple but profoundly powerful formula.

Cue + Routine = Reward

This formula is so empowering because once you understand the three pieces involved in forming habits, you can start to move the pieces around to get different outcomes. It's just like playing chess, when you sit back from the chessboard and consider which moves to make in order to end up where you want to be. This information can help you become your own life coach. Your own therapist. Your own behavioral change agent who knows how to create the kinds of healthy habits that will lead to the success you want in your life.

Let's take a closer look at the formula for habits. The **cue** can be just about anything. The time of day. A physical sensation like hunger. A psychological desire, like the desire to feel accepted by others. A situation in your environment that you want to change, like wanting a clean desk instead of a messy desk. The cue creates a desire in you to do something. It acts as a trigger that causes you to feel motivated to respond. Whatever you are motivated to do becomes your **routine** or response to the event. In strict psychological terms, the cue is called a **stimulus**, and the routine is called a **response**, as proposed by behavioral scientist, B.F. Skinner.

You are likely to keep repeating your routine if it is followed by a **reward.** The reward can be an internal reward, like feeling happy. The reward can also be an external reward, like when people seem to approve of your response. If you keep repeating this routine and keep getting a reward for it, eventually it will become a habit, something you do automatically without conscious thought. Let's look at these examples.

Cue: You feel hungry.
Routine: You eat something.
Reward: You feel satisfied and no longer hungry.

Cue: You want to feel accepted by others.
Routine: You do things you think will please others (like wearing certain clothes).
Reward: Others tell you they like your response (they compliment you on your clothes), which makes you feel accepted by others and happy with yourself.

Cue: Your messy desk is annoying.
Routine: You clean off your desk.

Reward: You feel more comfortable and no longer annoyed.

As you can see from these examples, the routines that become habits usually have more than one reward. When your response to feeling hungry is to eat something, you feel satisfied, which is a form of pleasure. And when you eliminate the hunger sensation, it removes a source of discomfort, which we often experience as a form of pain. So responses are often rewarded by helping you find pleasure and avoid pain, which is the basic motivation for all human behavior. I can't tell you how powerful it is when you learn how to *use* this primal motivation to your advantage to change your daily habits.

Charles Duhigg wrote a book called *The Power of Habit* which stayed on the New York Times Bestseller list for sixty weeks (yes, sixty). Duhigg included the formula for making and breaking habits that I just described. Clearly, that information met a need within his readers. In his book, Duhigg described his own experience of gaining weight, which sent him on a mission to find out how to change his habits and lose what he had gained. He tried several different behaviors and documented what happened after each one. In other words, he kept changing his routine or response, then looked for any reward(s) that followed each routine. After some trial and error, Duhigg found the winning combination of routines and rewards, and he easily lost the weight. That's the power of knowing how to move around the pieces of the habits formula until you get the outcome you want.

More specifically, here's what happened. Duhigg started by looking at any habits that had changed since he started gaining weight. He realized he had started eating a chocolate chip cookie when he was at work. By recognizing this new habit, Duhigg was following his own advice for how to change a habit, which consists of four steps.

Step 1: Identify the routine
The first step is to identify the routine. Duhigg completed this step when he realized his unhealthy routine happened around 3:30 each afternoon. He would get up from his desk, walk to the cafeteria in his office building, buy a cookie, socialize with a coworker or friend for about 10 minutes, then go back to his office.

Step 2: Experiment with rewards
The next step is to try different rewards for your routine. Here, you're not trying to change the routine but to simply understand what will satisfy your urge to get the cookie. Using Duhigg's habit as an example, you might

wonder if you just needed a quick break from work, so instead of walking to the cafeteria, you could take a short walk outside. In case you're hungry, you could go to the cafeteria and buy something else, like an apple, then eat it while socializing with a coworker. Keeping the rest of your routine the same, you could try drinking a cup of coffee instead of eating a cookie in case you're wanting an energy boost. Or you could simply take a break to talk with a friend.

Once you get back to your desk after experimenting with each reward, then wait fifteen minutes and write down how you feel. This will help you tune into the effects of each reward. For example, if you wanted an energy boost, give the caffeine in the coffee time to kick in. Then write down three words about how you feel. After fifteen minutes, let's say you feel energized, focused, and not hungry. Writing down how you feel will help you remember and analyze the results of each experiment.

This second step could take a few days to a few weeks, but it will be well worth your time and effort. By doing these experiments, Duhigg figured out he wasn't hungry and he wasn't seeking an energy boost. Instead, he wanted the reward of a temporary distraction, which he could get by talking with a friend.

Step 3: Isolate the cue
What started Duhigg's habit of going to the cafeteria? What was the cue that set off his routine? In this step, look for seven possible cues: **location** (sitting at your desk), **time** (3:30 p.m.), your **emotional state** (for example, bored), **other people** (no one else around), and any **immediately preceding actions** (just finished reviewing a report). Duhigg doesn't say this, but also look for a **physical sensation** (like thirst) or a **psychological desire** (like wanting connection with others). Do this for several days, write down what you observe, and see what patterns emerge. After analyzing the cues for three days, Duhigg could easily see that the only constant cue was the time of day. His weight-gaining routine was triggered between 3:00 – 4:00 p.m.

Step 4: Have a Plan
After you have identified the unhealthy routine, you have experimented to figure out the reward, and you know what cue triggers your routine, you're ready to plan for a new routine. In this step, you decide on a new routine that will give you the reward you want. Here's what Duhigg decided: *At 3:30, every day, I will walk to a friend's desk and talk for ten minutes.* He

even set an alarm on his watch to remind him to practice his new routine. Some days he was too busy to take a break. Some days it felt like too much effort to find someone who was available to talk, so he gave into the urge to buy the cookie. This type of backsliding is to be expected when you're establishing a new habit. But after a few weeks, Duhigg's new habit became automatic. Each day he successfully completed his new routine, he went home from work feeling a sense of accomplishment, which provided more rewards for his efforts.

Going through the four steps that Duhigg suggests can take a month or longer, but once you understand the three parts of your bad habit—the cue, routine, and reward—and after you have analyzed each one, you gain power over your old habit. It no longer controls you like it did. You are also prepared to create a healthy habit to take its place.

If you follow Duhigg's formula for changing a habit, you're almost guaranteed to succeed. You may also succeed by simply replacing your unhealthy habit with one that's healthy instead. Sometimes this can be a shortcut that works, especially if you visualize your success with lots of emotional enthusiasm. And especially if you also start to see yourself as the kind of person who already has the healthy habit you want to create. In other words, change your identity to help change your habit. Any of the other strategies for changes habits that are described in this chapter may also provide shortcuts from what Duhigg suggests. Just be aware your new habit may be harder to maintain if you don't identify the reward(s) for your old habit and find healthy substitutes for those rewards.

I want to mention one more important point about the last piece in the habits formula, the reward piece. Here's a heads up. Whether you're aware of it or not,

Every habit you have is being rewarded by dopamine.

That's right. All of your habits—your good habits and your not-so-good habits—have a reward or payoff of dopamine. As much as you might dislike or even despise a particular habit you have, you're getting some kind of a reward out of doing it, even if it's an unconscious reward. Otherwise, you wouldn't keep doing it. And that reward always includes dopamine. This feel-good brain chemical is hardwired into our brains to help us survive. According to Loretta Breuning, author of *Habits of a Happy Brain*, "You are designed to survive by seeking happy chemicals (in your brain) and avoiding unhappy chemicals." For example, dopamine keeps us searching for food because we have learned that eating will provide a reward for our hunger. It makes us feel good before we eat—when we *anticipate* eating— and when we do things to move toward getting something to eat. That means all our responses to the event of feeling hungry that involve moving toward food give us the energy and excitement that dopamine provides, *all along the way*. It motivates us to keep going. The same thing is true for all our responses when we anticipate they will lead us to a reward. Once you start to factor dopamine into your efforts to change your habits, things get a whole lot easier.

Why do they get easier? Because you can add more feel-good rewards to your efforts to change your habits, both after you establish your new habit and as you are moving toward that change. For example, I use both online and paper calendars. Keeping up with my hardcopy, paper calendar can be tedious. But I love certain colors, so I buy brightly colored calendars and use colored felt tip markers, which help me enjoy using my calendar much more. I decorate and organize my office and desk in ways that make me feel good. I keep motivational quotes where I will see them often. In other words, I set up my work environment in ways that tilt the Outer Game factors in my favor. I also give myself rewards for establishing new healthy habits that are part of my Inner Game or mindset. These rewards help me keep my thoughts and emotions positive. Rewards like lots and lots of positive self-talk—while I'm learning new habits and after they are established. All these rewards bring more dopamine and more good feelings.

What do you enjoy? What makes you feel good? Use that information to add more rewards into your efforts to change your habits and see what happens. Consider Outer Game and Inner Game rewards you could incorporate. In other words, sit back from the chessboard and see what moves or small rewards you can use that will help you build your new habits. As before, be careful about using rewards that involve food or spending money, because both of those can lead to problems.

What Habits Do You Want to Start? And What Habits Do You Want to Stop?

Napoleon Hill said, "A goal is a dream with a deadline." That's because our goals are finite. They have an end date, a completion time of when the goal is done. You finish your goal and move on to another goal. In contrast, habits are ongoing goals. They are goals you want to keep doing, sometimes indefinitely. For example, I want to keep the goal of getting enough quality sleep at night as a habit I have for the rest of my life.

Just like with limiting beliefs, you can outgrow your habits, and they can become **limiting habits** that no longer work. Habits that might have helped you get safely and successfully to where you are right now may not be able to take you into a new level of achievement in your future. It may take a while to realize that a habit that always worked before doesn't work now, so be on the lookout for outgrown habits if you keep trying to use a habit that doesn't help the way it used to.

For example, I used to stop exercising when I got extra busy because I didn't want to take time away from what I needed to get done. And that habit worked at the time. But now that I'm busier than ever, I need my workouts even more. I may not do my full exercise routine every time, but I've made it a habit to exercise every day, even if it's just working out to a five-minute online exercise video. I've outgrown my habit to stop exercising altogether, because I've learned over and over again that the time I spend exercising helps me get more things done, do them more quickly, and feel better as I'm doing them.

To take full advantage of the information you will learn in this chapter, I suggest you start by identifying what habits you want to start doing and which ones you want to stop doing. Go back to where you're keeping your writing for this book and quickly write down two lists. One list is habits to start. The other list is habits to stop. Don't overthink your responses. Just write down whatever comes into your mind. You may find that some of your habits are also on the lists of goals you wrote down earlier. That's fine. It probably just means those are goals you want to turn into habits and keep doing indefinitely.

Once you have your two lists, then give yourself another few minutes to look over the lists to see if there's anything you want to change on either list. Maybe add or delete one or more of the habits you wrote down? When you feel comfortable with both lists, then take another minute to consider what one habit you either want to start or stop doing right now. You may want to choose this as your **practice habit** as you go through the rest of this chapter. But before you make a final decision on your practice habit, read through this next section on prioritizing the habits you want to change.

How to Prioritize Which Habits You Start and Stop

Most of us can come up with long lists of habits we want to change. But we can't change all of them at once, so we need to prioritize. You can choose whatever you want for your practice habit, but some habits are better to start with than others. The following information gives you a few considerations for prioritizing.

1. Pick a habit that is small and easy.
With this suggestion, you want to choose a habit that is so small and so easy that it won't take you out of your comfort zone and may even be something you would enjoy. Or pick a more difficult habit to change, then break it into such small steps that you're almost guaranteed to succeed at each one. For example, if you want to lose weight, you could start by eating off of a smaller plate to help control your portion sizes. Or you could put your fork down in between bites to help you eat slower.

Or let's say you want to make it a habit to spend more time with your family. Take one small step toward developing that habit by simply asking one of your family members what that person would enjoy doing together. Be sure to offer your own suggestions, like going out to eat or to a movie. The next step might be to spend time together doing something you enjoy, say once a month. Then gradually increase the activities and frequency of your together time. Many married couples have regular "date nights" to make sure they have quality time together. I suggest you schedule your activities on your calendar to help make them a priority. When you're successful with small and easy habits, it gives you the confidence and motivation to want to change more of them.

2. Pick a habit that gives you the greatest gains.
Another way to prioritize which habits to work on first is to consider which habits would provide the most mileage for your efforts. In other words, which habits would give you the greatest gains if you were to put those habits in place? This quote by Tony Robbins offers a suggestion:

What's the most important factor to creating a extraordinary life? The answer is energy.

That's right, energy. Healthy habits can transform your life, but changing your habits takes energy. If you develop and maintain daily habits that improve your health, those habits will help give you the energy to create more healthy habits and do other things you want to do in your life.

Decades of research have shown that improving your health in three areas can provide a foundation for natural energy and abundant health: diet, sleep, and exercise. I've found that if I maintain healthy habits in these three areas, the rest of my life is much easier and more enjoyable. I'm better able to handle the day-to-day stressors that come along, deal with the obstacles and setbacks that are a normal part of life, and have enough energy to achieve more challenging goals. Plus, I'm in a good mood most of the time. But I will say, I work at it. I understand that my health is the foundation for a successful life. Without your health, it's hard to enjoy much of anything else.

I can't encourage you enough to stop your unhealthy habits. Most people can quickly boost their energy levels by changing a few key bad habits like these examples that people have shared with me. Stop staying up so late at night. Get off the junk food. Cut out the sodas and sugary drinks. Stop drinking too much alcohol. Turn off the TV and stop sitting for so long. Put down your phone and stop staring at your screen for hours every day. And here are some healthy habits you might want to start. Get seven to eight hours of sleep at night. Eat more unprocessed foods like fruits and vegetables. Find a way to exercise regularly, even when you don't want to. Decide this is the best time to get serious about taking care of your health. Because it is.

The information in the rest of this chapter will give you strategies and suggestions on how to change unhealthy habits. However, please understand that it's hard enough to change your habits when you're healthy and feeling good. It's much harder if you're sleep deprived, feeding your brain and body junk food, and not recharging your energy levels with exercise. Remember: when surveyed, the number one reason people gave for why they procrastinate was because of fatigue, because they were "too tired." But just to clarify, the research by Piers Steel clearly shows that the main cause of procrastination is impulsiveness. Although this may seem contradictory, it actually makes sense when you consider that fatigue can make you more impulsive. When you're tired, you are more likely to impulsively do what feels good and what's easiest, even when that means procrastinating on what you need to get done. In other words, you do what is easiest in the moment, even if it involves an unhealthy habit.

3. Pick whatever habit feels right to start with.

Some people are bored by making small changes in their habits. Instead, they feel more motivated if they start with major habits like running a successful business or getting and staying physically fit. That's fine as long as you break your habits into small enough steps to avoid getting overwhelmed. Or sometimes certain habits we have bother us more than others. We may feel bad about ourselves for having that habit, or other people may tell us our habit bothers them. For example, checking your phone when you're in a conversation with someone else can make that person feel ignored, disrespected, and annoyed. It's called **phubbing,** or phone snubbing, and it can damage your relationships faster than you might think. A good place to start changing this habit might be to adopt a rule of "No phones at the table" when you're eating meals with others. If your phone is out of sight, and if your notifications are turned off during mealtime, you might get some quick success on breaking one aspect of this habit.

How Many and How Long?

Before we get into specific strategies for changing habits, I want to answer the two most frequent questions I get from people about how to start and stop them.

How many habits should you try to change at one time?

This question is one I often get from people related to how many goals they should take on at the same time. The answer to that question is that *it depends*. It depends on the person, on the goal or habit they want to change, on the amount of internal resistance to that change, along with several other factors. But since habits are just ongoing goals, here's my suggestion for both. Start out with no more than three goals or habits you want to change all at once. See how you do. If you get early success with all three, that number may be fine. But it you're struggling with as many as three habits, cut back to no more than one or two and keep your attention squarely on those until they become automatic. Then pick another goal or habit to work on and focus on that until you either complete the goal or form a new habit.

How long does it take to change a habit?

You may have heard it takes twenty-one days to change a habit. In some cases, and for some people, I think that's true, give or take a little time depending on what the habit is. More recent research suggests that on average it takes 66 days to change a habit. For the group of people in the study, that was the average of how long it took.

There is also the possibility of what's called **one-shot learning**, where you establish a new habit the first time you do it. I know people who were diagnosed with a serious illness and managed to change a lot of habits practically overnight. Obviously, their motivation level was high. A number of times, I have personally changed small habits with just one try. For instance, if I want to start taking a new vitamin, I will keep the vitamin bottle out on my kitchen counter as a visual reminder to take it every day, and that usually works. Once I have established the habit of taking it, I can put the bottle away, somewhere out of sight. You can also use the alarm and reminders functions on your phone until a new habit takes hold.

In my many years of helping people with goal setting and habit change, I have found that just like how many goals you can change all at once *depends*, how long it takes to change a habit also *depends*. It depends on a lot of factors, like how important the new habit is, how much experience the person has with changing habits, whether their underlying beliefs are limiting or empowering, and whether they have support from others. It depends.

The key point for me is that I don't want to pre-program my conscious mind or my subconscious mind to expect that it will take 21 days, or 66 days, or however long someone else tells me it will take to change a habit. It may not take that long at all. The message here is to continue to move toward establishing the new habit **as long as it takes** for it to become automatic. Please don't get it in your head that it will take you a certain amount of time to change a habit. Give 100 percent to your effort and be open to the possibility that you can establish new habits faster than you might expect.

Also, here's some exciting news about how long it takes to change your habits. In her book *Habits of a Happy Brain,* Loretta Breuning says that because of the way our brains are wired, there are two ways we learn: (1) **repetition**, which helps us learn gradually and (2) **emotion**, which can cause us to learn something instantly. I'll never forget talking with the head coach of a successful college football team. His mantra was "Seven repetitions." That's how many times it took for his players to learn their drills well enough to perform them under the pressure of an important football game.

In contrast, people who are diagnosed with a serious illness often react with strong emotions, which can help them learn new habits almost instantly. This type of emotionally charged situation can result in one-shot learning. Another example? People who have experienced some type of trauma may learn something instantly. If you're in a serious car accident, you may immediately learn to become a better defensive driver. Your strong emotions immediately change the wiring in your brain. That's one of the reasons why the imagery used with sport psychology works so well, because it includes seeing, hearing, and *feeling* the success of whatever you want to achieve. I highly recommend you use this type of imagery to help change your habits faster and easier. Remember to feel the emotions of your success for about thirty seconds. You can use the imagery along with any of the other techniques in this chapter that you decide to try.

Here's the Bottom-Line Question

If you haven't already, right now make your final choice about your practice habit, something you want to either start or stop doing. It might be easy to change that habit and it might not take that long. Or it might be harder to change that habit and it might take longer than you hoped. Either way, commit to sticking with it until you're successful. But because some habits can be so stubborn and difficult to change, here's the bottom-line question for all of us:

How do you make yourself do things you don't want to do?

If you're a chronic procrastinator and you want to get serious about overcoming it, your first answer to that question might be that you look for quick fixes, like some of the Outer Game strategies on goal setting and time management. But you may have already found those usually don't work, at least not for long. Instead, I suggest that you address the 80-plus percent of Inner Game obstacles that are created by your fears and limiting beliefs. In other words, get out of your own way and stop sabotaging your own efforts. Hopefully, you have already done at least some of that by using the techniques in earlier parts of this book. Techniques like finding a happy ending to your procrastination story (Chapter Three), nudging yourself out of your comfort zone (Chapter Three), outsmarting impulsiveness (Chapter Four), and transforming your limiting beliefs into empowering ones (Chapter Five).

If you are still struggling to make yourself do things you don't want to do, just know that you're not alone. We all struggle at times. But in order not to stay stuck in that struggle, I encourage you to keep experimenting with different strategies until you find what works. Like Charles Duhigg, keep trying different responses and different rewards until you discover which pieces of the habit formula will add up to the correct combination. Become intensely curious about finding at least one strategy that will get you past your resistance for long enough to establish a new habit. Compared to the benefits you will gain by having your new habit, it won't take that long. You'll look back at the time it took to change that habit and be so grateful you hung in there until the new habit became automatic.

But remember this quote from Jen Sincero: "In order to kick ass you must first lift up your foot." If you want something to change, you will need to *do something* to get started. That something can be as simple as rewarding your brain with dopamine. This will add positive emotions to your efforts because dopamine makes us feel happy and excited, which can help us learn faster. Imagining how good you will feel after you establish a new habit will give your brain a shot of dopamine. Visualizing what your future success will look like will trigger a dopamine reward. You'll also get a surge of dopamine when you're actively searching for the winning combination of the pieces in the habits formula. Discovering what techniques *don't* work can also release the good feelings that dopamine provides, because that means you're one step closer to finding what *does* work. So do something—even if it's just visualizing your success or trying a technique that doesn't work. Dopamine, and the emotions it creates, will kick in and help you keep going.

With all of the suggestions and strategies in this chapter, if you think a particular habit will be especially challenging, I encourage you to first go back to Chapter Six on goals and write down a Plan for Success and a Plan for Failure. The few minutes it will take you to write out your plans can make all the difference in whether you succeed, so I encourage you to give yourself this extra advantage. As we covered before, just writing down the goal you want to achieve can boost your odds of success by 39.5 percent. And writing to a friend about your progress stacks the odds of success in your favor by an extraordinary 76.7 percent. These same techniques also work with habits. Set things up at the beginning of your efforts so the odds are in your favor. And throughout this chapter, keep in mind that it's usually not about adding more time or more habits into your day. It's about replacing any current habits that are not supporting your future success. Once you develop the right habits and do them daily, your life will never be the same.

Shortcuts for Changing Your Habits

Besides tapping into dopamine at the beginning of my efforts, I have found several shortcuts for changing habits that I want to describe here. I'll suggest additional techniques after that. But sometimes these shortcuts are all you need to either start or stop a habit, so they might be worth a little experimenting to see if that's the case for you. Read through this list. Pick the one you think would be the most likely to work. Give it a sincere, good-faith effort and notice what happens. Write down the results. Let your results speak for themselves.

1. Change Your Environment

As we covered before, sometimes the quickest and easiest way to change your behavior is to make changes in the Outer Game factors—in your environment. In general, you want to set up your environment in ways that support your goals and good habits and help you break bad habits. In other words, **make it easy to do the right thing and hard to do the wrong thing**. This may be as simple as getting rid of distractions and clutter in your house and workspace. Make it a habit to keep the clutter out of your life from now on. Or let's say you want to create a habit of walking first thing in the morning. Place your walking clothes out the night before so they will be ready to put on when you first get up.

If you often forget where you left your keys when you come in your house, decide on one place where you will keep them. Maybe on a special wall peg or in a tray on your bedroom dresser. Designate a place and make it a habit to keep them there. You could even put a note in that place that says "Keys" until you get in the habit of using it. Or if your children have gotten into the bad habit of taking their phones into their bedrooms at night and staying up too late because they're on social media, maybe you could get a phone charger with multiple ports, keep it on the kitchen counter, and make it a rule that all phones stay on the counter once it's time for bed. A friend of mine did this and found that her children protested at first but eventually got used to it when she held firm on the new rule. Plus, her kids became more accepting when they started feeling better because they were getting more sleep.

Here's another example. In general, I eat a healthy diet and don't crave any particular foods. But cashews are my downfall. A few cashews are fine, but once I start eating them, I can't seem to stop. They are so high in fat that too many cashews can zap my energy and make me feel sick to my stomach. But I will still eat more than I should and end up feeling nauseous, with practically no energy.

What I've observed about this habit is that if I buy the cashews and have them in my house, it sets me up for an argument in my head, a mental tug-of-war that can become louder and more distracting over time. The inner battle of thoughts in my head include things like *I want to eat some cashews now,* followed by thoughts that say *You better not. You know you can't stop.* Those kinds of thoughts can take over my mental airways, drawing my attention away from whatever I'm trying to do. Usually, the outcome of that argument is that I get tired and worn down by the internal fighting, and I give in to the thoughts to eat the cashews just to get the fighting to stop. Then the pattern repeats: I eat too many, I feel sick, and I feel bad about myself for not being able to control my behavior.

I've found that the quickest and easiest way to avoid this whole internal drama is to not buy the cashews in the first place. If I change my environment and remove the temptation so it's no longer readily available, I no longer have the problem. I won't leave my house to go buy cashews if I notice a craving. I simply eat something else I already have at home, and the craving and conflicting thoughts quickly disappear.

2. Shift Your Identity

For a while, I watched a lot of YouTube videos that teach you shortcuts on how to keep your house decluttered, organized, and clean. I found one called "3 Little Habits that Changed my Life" by Kallie Branciforte. In that video, Branciforte describes how she struggled with her house always being messy and found it difficult to change her bad habits. She had read

James Clear's bestselling book, *Atomic Habits,* where he suggests shifting your identity as a way of changing your habits, and Branciforte decided to try it. She started thinking of herself as a tidy person instead of a messy person, and almost immediately, she found it easier to adopt the habits that would keep her house in order. An identity shift helps to transform our core limiting beliefs about ourselves and can provide a shortcut to creating positive new habits. Our new habits reinforce our new identity and make it easier to maintain that shift in the long run.

I've made several identity shifts with my procrastination. I've gone from an **always-running-late** kind of person, to a **barely-on-time** kind of person, to an **easily-on-time** person, to an **ahead-of-time** person. Each shift has made me feel more empowered. I can't believe how much better I feel about myself now and how much less stress I have in my life. What about you? Try thinking about yourself as an easily-on-time person or an ahead-of-time person and see if that makes it easier for you to establish habits of doing things sooner than you used to.

In case you're interested, here's why this strategy works. Your brain is constantly seeking to make sense of your experiences, and it wants congruence between who you think you are as a person (your core identity) and how you think and act. If you think and act differently than what you believe to be your core identity, it creates something called **cognitive dissonance**, which causes stress. For example, if you think of yourself as a responsible person and you do something that is irresponsible, it will bother you and you will feel uncomfortable, which is a source of stress. You can remove this stress by thinking and acting in ways that are aligned with your core beliefs. You can also use this function of your brain to your advantage by first shifting your identity so your habits naturally fall in line.

3. Question Your Beliefs About Why You Have a Bad Habit
Your thoughts and beliefs can cause you to hang onto a bad habit because you mistakenly think that habit is somehow beneficial. In other words, the payoffs or rewards you *think* you're getting from a bad habit may not be payoffs at all.

Probably the most effective book to help people stop smoking is one called *The Easy Way to Stop Smoking* by Allen Carr. This book has helped millions of people around the world put down their last cigarette and never smoke again. Nicotine is one of the most addictive substances there is, right up there with heroine. So how does simply reading a book help smokers quit?

Carr teaches readers what he learned when he quit his own 30-year addiction to smoking. He teaches them to question the beliefs they have around why they need to smoke in the first place. For example, smokers often think *I enjoy smoking too much to give it up,* and *If I quit, I'm afraid I will always feel deprived.* As you might imagine, these beliefs create a fear of quitting, and that fear, along with their limiting beliefs, form an inner block, a self-made obstacle that keeps them lighting up.

Throughout the book, Carr challenges smokers' limiting beliefs, and he hammers home the empowering beliefs that will help them quit. Through a combination of harsh reality, tough love, and empathic understanding, Carr says things like:

- Stop lying to yourself. You know you don't enjoy smoking. There's nothing enjoyable about being a slave to an addiction that could prematurely end your life.
- Until you quit, you're depriving yourself of your health, your money, your self-respect, your energy, your self-esteem, and your freedom.
- It won't be easier to quit tomorrow, because with drug addiction, you get progressively more hooked, not less.
- Just think of how wonderful it will be to not be controlled by your addiction and to instead be a happy non-smoker, enjoying the gifts of health, happiness, and freedom.

By the time readers have finished the book, they no longer believe their limiting thoughts and no longer have a fear of quitting. Instead, they have a new understanding and a new set of empowering beliefs about smoking. They are ready to successfully stop a habit they may have had most of their lives and never pick up another cigarette. Powerful stuff.

You can do the same thing with your own unhealthy habits. Pick one unhealthy habit and write down all the reasons why you might want to continue doing it. Even if your reasons seem unreasonable when you examine them, write them down anyway. Then write down empowering thoughts that will help break your bad habit. Whenever you want to repeat your unhealthy habit, pause. Stop your automatic response. Remember why your unhealthy habit doesn't serve you. Review your list of empowering statements and let those statements help support your efforts to change.

You can also use this strategy with your procrastination in general. Write down all the reasons you might want to continue to procrastinate. Maybe things like *When I procrastinate, I get to avoid doing things I don't want to do, which makes me feel powerful and in control.* Then write down positive statements that include a reality check and some tough love. Things like *Are you kidding? You know your procrastination inevitably leads to missed opportunities, being mad at yourself, and feeling out of control.* Read through your list of empowering statements when you're tempted to put things off. Make sure your tough love statements do not include any self-criticism, blaming, or shaming. Just straightforward and honest facts.

4. Identify the Rewards for Your Bad Habit

One of the fastest ways I know to stop a bad habit is to focus in on the last piece of the habits formula—on the rewards you're getting for your response. Besides dopamine, figure out the payoff or reward and find healthy ways to get that same payoff. In the first chapter of this book, I told the story of how being late to meetings at work was damaging my professional reputation. I couldn't seem to change my bad habit until I realized that I was getting a reward for my behavior. Being late made me feel powerful. Once I found healthy ways to feel powerful, I could more easily start getting to meetings on time. Sometimes, just figuring out what reward you're getting for your bad habit is enough to help you break that habit and start doing something else. It can be a quick fix that is surprisingly simple to do.

If you want to break a bad habit, then right now, ask yourself, "What is the payoff for my behavior?" Often, you will be getting more than one reward. Being late to meetings not only made me feel powerful, it also provided a kind of intensity in my life that helped keep me from feeling bored. So I started getting really good at my job and challenged myself to do everything in my life on time. That change helped me feel challenged and powerful in healthy ways and kept me from feeling bored. Plus, I got dopamine rewards from my brain after each small success and during all my efforts to change.

5. Replace a Bad Habit with a Good One

If you try to stop a bad habit without replacing it with another activity or habit, you create a void that usually gets filled with anxiety. This anxiety makes it more likely you will quickly fall back into your old habit. It's better to find something you can substitute for the habit you want to break. Chew nicotine gum or use a skin patch instead of smoking cigarettes. Squeeze a stress ball instead of biting your fingernails. Replace soda with water or a healthy sports drink. Instead of snacking on junk food, find healthy snacks that are convenient and easy to carry around. Find a fun project and work on that in your spare time instead of watching too much TV. If you want to stop being so self-critical, use a journal to identify your negative thoughts and self-talk and replace those with positive affirmations. The point is to substitute an unhealthy habit with one that is healthy, or at least healthier than what you were doing. And make the healthier habit as easy and as convenient as you can.

6. Reward Yourself for Effort

Find ways to motivate yourself by using rewards, even if it's just self-talk that says, "Good job. Way to go. You're doing great. Keep at it. You've got this." Reward yourself even if your efforts haven't been perfect. And perhaps especially reward yourself if your efforts made you uncomfortable. Avoid comparisons to other people and how well they may be doing. Stay focused on running your own race. You're only competing against yourself. Your only goal is to be better than you were yesterday, last week, last month, last year. Any progress is progress. The more you can reward yourself for your efforts, the more dopamine will help you keep going.

And please have some compassion for yourself when you make mistakes, get sidetracked, and run into dead ends. Hey. At least you're in the game. Getting some scrapes and bruises is to be expected when you're on the playing field. It's much better than sitting on the sidelines and not going after what you want. So get into a habit of using compassionate and encouraging self-talk, especially when your efforts don't help you succeed right away.

Here's what doesn't work, at least not for long. Punishment. Punishment may deter problem behavior temporarily but it usually doesn't lead to lasting change. It can make you shut down, strip away your sense of empowerment, and make you passive and submissive. You may end up feeling helpless and hopeless. The reason treats are used to train animals is because rewards work so much better than punishment. You give a treat to your dog after it does what you want it to do. This is called **positive reinforcement** because it reinforces the behavior you want your dog to repeat. The same principle works with people.

Unfortunately, many people go through their whole lives using self-punishment techniques like criticism, guilt trips, blaming, shaming, and imposing unreasonable restrictions and expectations. It's probably because that's how they were raised. But they never acknowledge to themselves that these types of punitive techniques rarely, if ever, help them change their behavior in the long run or get the results they want. Which means they never have the chance to learn healthier and more effective ways of motivating themselves to change.

If this situation applies to you, ask yourself this simple question: "Do my guilt trips and self-punishment help me succeed?" That question could be all it takes to start finding different techniques for self-motivation, ones that actually will work. Additional questions to ask include, "If punishment doesn't work when I do something 'wrong,' what are some healthy rewards I can use when I do things that are 'right?'" Try rewarding your positive behavior instead of punishing whatever you consider negative behavior. Then observe what happens.

There's one additional downside to punishment and excessive guilt. As we covered before in Chapter Four, our Inner Child includes a Party Child who doesn't want to be told "No." If you are unreasonable with your restrictions and expectations, this Party Child will often rebel and create havoc in your life. You may have experienced times in your life when this happened. The time you went on that crazy restrictive diet, lost weight, then quickly gained it all back, plus some extra pounds. The time you expected yourself to work too long and hard, then sat on your couch and binge watched Netflix movies for the next two days. The main takeaway here is that using positive rewards and setting reasonable expectations will give you the best chances for success.

I want to also mention, though, that there's an upside to guilt. We usually feel guilty when we think we have violated our own moral or ethical standards. Let's say you unintentionally hurt someone else, and now you feel guilty. When we respond to this kind of guilt in positive ways, it can motivate us to take responsibility for our mistakes, learn the lessons from our experiences, and not repeat them in the future. In this example, your guilt may be a message that you need to apologize to that person and promise not to hurt them again, which is a good thing. After you apologize and learn your lessons, the guilt usually goes away. However, many procrastinators don't respond to guilt in positive ways. Instead, they constantly make themselves feel guilty for what they perceive as their own wrongdoings against themselves or others, usually through their self-talk. They don't learn their lessons, and they keep repeating the same mistakes. Their guilt becomes excessive and prolonged, and it can lead to anxiety, depression, and low self-esteem.

I encourage you to become more aware of when your thoughts are making you feel guilty. Understand it's possible that your guilt may be due to a mistake or wrongdoing that you need to correct. If that's the case, take responsibility for your mistake and learn what it has to teach.

7. Use the Peace Process

If you get stuck when you try to change a particular habit, use the Peace Process (see Chapter Five). Sometimes our bad habits and our resistance to building good habits are caused by emotions that are trapped in our bodies. For example, a woman who lost a substantial amount of weight and managed to keep it off for many years, put it something like this: "I had a trapped feeling inside of me, and I tried to use food to make it go away. Once I identified the problem that was causing the feeling, I stopped using food to try to fix it and easily lost the weight."

This is a common habit. Many people are emotional overeaters. They overeat to numb their uncomfortable feelings instead of dealing with the feelings and with whatever is making them feel uncomfortable in the first place. In their defense, these people probably don't know what else to do with these emotions. They keep overeating because they don't know of any other options. The same is often true with many addictions. We turn to our addictions when we don't want to feel what we're feeling, and we simply don't know of any alternatives to make the feelings go away. For example, Bill Wilson, co-founder of Alcoholics Anonymous (AA), believed that buried feelings often result in alcoholism and that the primary emotion that contributes to alcoholism is resentment.

On top of that, we often develop limiting beliefs which tell us that numbing our bad feelings is the *only* way to get rid of them. **This is how our emotions can result in limiting beliefs, and why releasing the emotions FIRST can be the best way to deal with the emotions and the beliefs.** You may remember from earlier in this book, this is what psychiatrist David Hawkins says in his book, *Letting Go*. It is probably why he got such good results with his patients. Release the bad feelings first, and the unhealthy thoughts and beliefs around those bad feelings will naturally fall away. This is a huge piece of the therapeutic puzzle.

Here's Why the Peace Process Works

Recent discoveries in brain research have shown exactly *why* mind-body techniques help people release negative emotions. These techniques include the Peace Process, Tapping (sometimes called Emotional Freedom Technique or EFT), Neuro Emotional Technique (NET), Eye Movement Desensitization and Reprocessing (EMDR), hypnosis, the RIM Method (Regenerative Images in Memory), and visualization which focuses on the body. One of the early pioneers in this field was Bernie Siegel, a surgeon specializing in cancer treatment. In his book *Love, Medicine and Miracles*, Siegel reports the miraculous healings that people in his cancer research studies were able to obtain by using medical treatments along with visualizing the healing that was happening inside their bodies. The participants in his studies were often those who had been told their cancer was terminal because standard medical treatments hadn't worked. In almost every case, patients could identify a traumatizing experience that happened right before they got their cancer diagnosis, which no doubt led to lots of negative emotions.

According to Loretta Breuning, author of *Habits of a Happy Brain*, "Emotions are chemical molecules . . . (in the body)." Whoa. Just by itself, that definition of emotions gives us a clue that mind-body techniques might help us manage them. But then, get this.

In her international bestselling book *Goodbye, Hurt and Pain*, Dr. Deborah Sandella, a therapist and originator of the RIM Method, describes exactly *how* feelings get trapped in our bodies. Here's what she writes. "(Strong emotions) . . . create a biochemical event that automatically anchors in body memory." She adds, "The greater the emotional intensity of an event, the more strongly the feelings get stuck in the nervous system. Strong feelings create a biochemical change, and when highly charged (negatively or positively), they gain immense stickiness in the body. In contrast, neutral experiences are easily forgotten." Sandella also explains that "The longer an issue has been underground, the stickier it grows. It takes on a life of its own that is outside the influence of the logical mind, which makes us feel out-of-control and anxious."

So what's going on here? Our strong emotions create a biochemical change that is "sticky" and can get stuck in the body. When we acknowledge and accept these emotions, they have a short life. They don't get stuck and they don't stay around very long. The sensation of the feelings and the chemical reactions they create come and go quickly—within minutes—*IF* we don't block them from our conscious awareness and refuse to accept them. But when we repress our feelings and deny we have them, both the chemicals and the emotions that cause them get stuck somewhere in our bodies and stay there. The positive feelings that get stored in our bodies are usually not a problem. It's the negative emotions that can create a lifetime of problems if they are not released. Because here's the deal.

What You Resist Persists

There's a well-known quote by the Swiss psychiatrist Carl Jung that says, "What you resist persists." That is definitely the case when it comes to resisting our feelings. Our unaccepted and unexpressed feelings don't just lay low and stay quiet. According to Sigmund Freud, the Austrian neurologist who founded psychoanalysis, "Unexpressed emotions will never die. They are buried alive and come forth later in uglier ways." Those uglier ways can include all kinds of mental health issues like anxiety and depression and all kinds of physical health problems. As Bernie Siegel found, these buried emotions may even be related to cancer.

Besides mental and physical health problems, do you know what else these buried emotions can cause? Yep. Procrastination. Especially chronic procrastination. We know from the definition of procrastination that we avoid doing things that make us feel uncomfortable. Whether that discomfort is fear, doubt, dread, anxiety, frustration, helplessness, or any other uncomfortable feelings, we put on the brakes when we go to do those things. **We're not avoiding the activity as much as the emotion that doing the activity makes us feel.**

Most of us already have an overload of negative feelings trapped inside of us from all the times in the past when we felt those emotions strongly but didn't accept and release them. We trigger that backlog of emotions from our past when we do something that makes us feel that same way in the present. Suddenly, the activity we want to do makes us feel completely overwhelmed with one or more negative emotions. That makes perfect sense when you consider all the sticky emotions that are already trapped inside. **The emotions get stuck in your body, then you get stuck in your life**. What you can't see is that the invisible feelings stuck inside of you are slamming on the brakes. The best way out of this bad habit is to release whatever emotions might be holding you back, then build the good habits that will help you move forward and keep going.

The findings reported by Sandella make even more sense when you add in what we covered earlier about how emotions can lead to the fastest learning. Repetition helps us learn, but emotions can help us learn even faster. As Loretta Breuning states, we can learn something instantly if is accompanied by strong emotions. When those strong emotions get trapped in the body, they make it not only easier to remember, but almost impossible to forget.

The strong negative emotions that stick around in our bodies play a protective role in our safety and survival. Trauma teaches. And intensely negative trauma teaches instantly. When it comes to negative and traumatic experiences, the sticky emotional and chemical reactions can do two things: **(1) they can keep you safe and (2) they can keep you stuck**. If you don't release the intense emotions that negative experiences create, they can cause all kinds of emotional blocks, which can lead to all kinds of problems in the present and in the future. We now know that mind-body techniques can help clear out these emotional blocks, along with the limiting beliefs they may have caused. Because they release these internal blocks, these techniques can open the door for us to do whatever activities have caused us to procrastinate.

The emotional chemicals that stick around in our bodies are what I mentioned earlier about emotional residue. Even after people have identified, accepted, and expressed their negative emotions, sometimes those emotions still cause them to get stuck in their lives because at that point it's not as much a psychological block as it is a biochemical block.

I'll never forget working with a chiropractor who practiced the Neuro Emotional Technique, where you clear emotions from the body by using certain acupressure points. I discovered a feeling that was trapped in my body. Based on neuromuscular testing, my chiropractor could tell I had done the therapeutic work to release the feeling on a psychological level. But the feeling was still trapped at the physical level, so we used the biological pressure points to release it from my body. I left her office feeling a remarkable lightness and freedom. Sometimes as with the Peace Process, the final and complete release of the emotion only takes a few minutes. Fascinating.

Bessel van der Kolk wrote a book called *The Body Keeps the Score* based on his experiences as a psychiatrist specializing in emotional trauma. His entire career has focused on helping people release the emotions that are trapped in their bodies. According to van der Kolk, self-awareness is at the core of recovery. Becoming more aware of our bodies helps us get in touch with our inner world. Simply noticing our emotions (in our bodies) helps us move past our automatic, habitual reactions. He further states that, "When we pay focused attention to our bodily sensations, we can recognize the ebb and flow of our emotions and, with that, increase our control over them." He then adds "Once you pay attention to your physical sensations, the next step is to label them, as in, 'When I feel anxious, I feel a crushing sensation in my chest.'"

What van der Kolk describes is almost identical to the steps in the Peace Process. What's so hopeful is that the Peace Process can lead to quick and dramatic results—without needing to know the exact emotions or the limiting beliefs that are associated with them. When you focus your attention on the place in your body where the emotion got trapped, your attention acts like a laser beam shining light on that emotion, helping to release the emotion and the chemicals it created. Your acceptance of that feeling and your focused attention on where it got stuck in your body can release emotions you may have been carrying around since you were a child, along with the limiting beliefs they may have caused.

This more recent knowledge that emotions get trapped in your body is now going mainstream. If you Google "trapped emotions in the body," you will find a growing field of information. Some of this information refers to it as "trauma" that gets stuck in the body, as is the case with many of the YouTube videos posted by therapists. With most of these techniques, including Tapping and the Peace Process, you can use them with yourself once you learn how—through personal instruction, online videos, or by reading a book. We are so fortunate right now. With this knowledge, we can use mind-body techniques to help heal ourselves and others. And it's all free. There's no cost except the time and effort involved.

The Sandy Hook Project

Here's an example of how these mind-body techniques can lead to quick and powerful results. Nick Ortner is the author of several books on Tapping, including *The Tapping Solution*. Ortner lived in Newtown, Connecticut in 2012 when the mass shooting happened at the elementary school there, Sandy Hook. He knew Tapping could help the people who were traumatized by the tragic deaths of the twenty-six children and adults who were killed. By setting up The Tapping Solution Foundation, Ortner was instrumental in teaching twenty local professionals how to do Tapping. In turn, those professionals taught it to the people who had been most affected by this event, including students, parents, school employees, and first responders.

Some of these people had been in traditional therapy for as long as a year, with minimal results, before they learned how to do Tapping. After eight to ten Tapping sessions, they reported that they felt essentially healed. If you want to watch a Facebook video where they describe their before-and-after experiences with Tapping, it's titled "Relief for Newtown, CT" and can be found if you google "Nick Ortner, Tapping, Sandy Hook." I also included a URL link in the Notes section at the back of this book.

By sharing this example, I'm not in any way criticizing or dismissing the effectiveness of traditional therapy. I have seen it result in remarkable healings and transformations, and it is the best choice for certain types of mental health issues. But as you can see from the testimonials of those in the video, when our emotions get stuck in our bodies, mind-body techniques can often lead to faster results.

More Strategies to Change Your Habits

I want to mention a few more of my favorite techniques for changing your habits. These techniques are often suggested in books on habits because they work well for a lot of people. A list of the books I'm most familiar with and that have been helpful for me is included in the Recommended Reading section. I encourage you to experiment with the following techniques and see what happens. If you need any additional incentive to give them a fair trial, consider this research finding by author Dawson Church,

People who meditate improved their ability to solve complex problems by 490 percent.

Can you imagine getting almost 500 percent better at solving the problems in your life? Just one technique could be all you need to establish a healthy habit like meditating. That one habit could help turn your life into the dream you want to live.

1. Make a Precommitment

We all like new beginnings. There's something special about starting new habits on New Year's Day. Special times can also include birthdays, anniversaries, graduations and when children are born. For example, I know several women who gave up caffeine when they became pregnant with their first child. Starting new habits on a special day can give those habits more meaning and importance. Decide on your start date well in advance. Give yourself time to mentally and emotionally adjust to that change in your life before you move into the action steps to make it happen. Write down a Plan for Success and a Plan for Failure for each habit you want to change.

2. Schedule It

Once you decide on a start date for your new habit, schedule it in your calendar. Whether it's a habit you plan to do every day, several times a week, or at any other time variable, scheduling a time when you do your habit will make it more likely to get done. You can make this technique even more effective if you also visualize yourself successfully completing your habit—*when you have it scheduled*— according to the sport psychology guidelines we covered at the end of Chapter Two. See your success. Hear it. Feel it. I like to do this type of imagery right before I go to sleep the night before I plan to start my new habit. When I get up the next morning, my brain is already programmed to succeed. I continue doing this nighttime imagery until my new habit becomes automatic. It seems to shorten the time that takes.

3. Use Habit Stacking

Another way to schedule a time to do your habit is called **habit stacking**. With this technique, you "stack" a new habit you want to start doing on top of another habit that is already established. For example, if you want to start drinking more water, drink a glass each morning right after you brush your teeth. If you want to become more grateful, think of one thing you're grateful for after you turn on your coffee maker. This technique can make it easier to start a new habit, because the already-established habit acts as the cue that starts your routine, so you have a built-in reminder.

4. Use the 1% Rule

There are two ways to use this technique.

- **Improve your life by 1% each day**. James Clear, author of *Atomic Habits*, suggests that you make it a habit to improve your life every day by 1%. If you do this for a year, by the end of that year you will end up thirty-seven times better than when you started. Wow.

  For example, if you want to get into the habit of exercising, improve your workouts by 1 percent every day. Maybe you start by walking around the block. Then you improve your exercise by 1 percent each day by learning how to walk farther. Then you improve by walking 1 percent faster each day. Then you slowly learn to run, farther and faster, keeping your improvements in the 1 percent zone. By the end of a year, you could probably run a marathon.

I like to use this technique by going the extra mile every day with my productivity. Maybe I get one extra chore done around the house than I normally would. Maybe I complete one small item on my to-do list that I wasn't planning to complete. Or perhaps I do a random act of kindness that will make a difference in someone else's life. None of my extra-mile activities are hard or take very long. But they give me a shot of dopamine at the time and make me feel good about myself at the end of the day.

- **Don't step more than 1 percent outside your comfort zone.** There's a second way you can use the 1% rule. Make small steps toward your new habit that are no more than 1 percent beyond what's normal and comfortable for you. This will help keep your subconscious mind from overreacting and thinking that you're leaving what's safe and heading into a danger zone. Once your subconscious sends out the alarms of danger and fear, it becomes harder to coax yourself into changing your habit. So take small steps in the direction of your new habit and go slowly. Do things that are easy and don't take much time.

For example, if you want to stop eating junk food, a small step in that direction might be to decide on one healthy food you could eat as a substitute. Next, you could buy that food when you're already shopping at the grocery store. Another small step might be to place your healthy food choice on your kitchen counter where you will be reminded it's available. The point is to find ways to slowly and steadily nudge yourself in the direction of your new habit. In contrast, if you were to go into your kitchen and throw out all your junk foods at the same time, you could trigger a fear response that would make it harder to eventually change your eating habits. For more information on this technique of taking small steps, see B.J. Fogg's book called *Tiny Habits*.

5. Write in a Journal

There are lots of ways you can use a journal to support your efforts to change your habits. Research shows that journaling is one of the quickest paths to self-awareness and gratitude. Journaling just three times a week can lead to tremendous personal growth. And you may only need to write down several sentences in order to get benefits. Do any of the following seem like ways of journaling that would be helpful for you?

- Use it as an **accountability journal**. At the end of each day, record your progress toward making and breaking the habits you're working on.
- Use it as an **awareness journal** to increase your awareness of what stops you from changing your habits. When you fail in your attempts to make or break a habit, write down what happened— what you wanted to do and what you did instead. Then write down what you could do differently the next time to increase your chances of success. When you are successful, write down what you did that worked.

You can also use an awareness journal to express your thoughts and emotions, especially about situations that are upsetting. Writing down what you're thinking and feeling can lead to clarity, and that clarity can help you find solutions to any problems you might have. If you don't want to express your emotions to another person, you can express them to yourself by writing them in your journal, which means you get them out and won't end up getting stuck with unexpressed feelings inside of yourself. Or you can write letters to people you're upset with, but never give those letters to them. Also, when you discover limiting thoughts and beliefs, use your journal to help change them into empowering statements and positive affirmations.

- Use it as an **outcomes journal**. I love this technique because it is so powerful. Think of one habit you want to either start or stop. Imagine what it will look like when you have successfully changed that habit. Write that down. Write down what that will sound like. And write down what that will feel like. Let yourself get into the feelings of your success and enjoy the experience of success before it happens. This is another way to do the sport psychology imagery, where you write down what you imagine success will be like. It can make you *want* to change your habits, because your new habits are already rewarding you with dopamine.

An additional strategy for breaking bad habits and building healthy ones is to identify the obstacles that are getting in the way. The next chapter explores one of the most common obstacles many of us face, so keep reading.

Whether you want to start a simple habit like flossing your teeth every day, or whether you want to stop a more difficult habit like smoking, the key to your success lies in being persistent. Keep experimenting. Keep trying different techniques until you find what works. Then stick with that technique for long enough for your behavior to become a habit. It might only take a short time for that to happen. Or it might take longer. But no matter how long it takes, your persistence will eventually lead to your success. Just don't stop.

Think of it this way. Changing your more difficult habits is like growing bamboo. This plant inspires me to be patient when I need to change a harder habit. That's because bamboo takes a long time to germinate in the ground. You plant the seeds, you water and nurture them every day, then you wait and wait and wait for what can seem like forever before you see the first sprouts. But once those sprouts pop up through the soil, they're off to the races. They grow faster and taller than any other plants. And once the roots are established, bamboo can spread into an incredibly abundant harvest.

That's the same way it is with our healthy habits. If you can be patient and keep going until your habits are well established and automatic, you get to reap the abundance of what your healthy habits produce. Vibrant energy and abundant health. Financial prosperity. Greater and greater levels of happiness. Studies show that the healthy habits of non-procrastinators help them reap all those rewards and more.

Just keep going.

Chapter 7 Highlights

Good job! You're on a roll. You've got this. You made it to the end of Chapter Seven, which means you're more than ahead of most book readers. You're obviously serious about overcoming your procrastination, you believe that's possible, and you're willing to put in the time and effort to make that happen. You definitely deserve congratulations.

We covered a lot in this chapter. If you can learn how to change your habits, you're halfway home to changing your life in all the ways you've wanted. When your healthy habits become automatic, your life will never be the same. Some people might see you as lucky. But what they don't see is that you have mastered the formula for changing habits so you can create your own "luck"—for the rest of your life. Here are some of the main points we covered.

1. Healthy habits are the foundation for a successful life. Learning how to make and break habits is more than worth your time.

2. Here's the formula for creating habits: **cue + routine = reward.** Based on psychological principles, this formula is so empowering because it allows you to experiment with the three parts in order to build the habits you want into your life.

3. Changing your habits takes energy. If you start by establishing healthy habits around your diet, sleep, and exercise, those will help give you the energy to create more healthy habits and do other things you want to do in your life.

Action Steps

Understanding how to establish healthy habits is the first step in building them into your daily routines. The second step is taking the imperfect and uncomfortable actions to learn what techniques work for you and stick with them long enough for your new routines to become automatic. Then your brain is free to learn more healthy habits. The opportunities are endless, and the rewards are extraordinary. Take these steps to make that happen.

1. Make two lists. One list is habits you want to start. The other is habits you want to stop.

2. Out of the habits you want to change, pick one **practice habit** based on the guidelines for how to prioritize which habits to change first.

3. Experiment with the shortcuts and techniques for changing habits. For example, change your environment, question your beliefs about why you have a bad habit, try habit stacking, and use the 1% rule. Let your results speak for themselves.

4. Be patient and persistent as you find which techniques will help you change your habits. Reward yourself for your efforts and trust that you will eventually succeed. Don't stop until you establish the habits you want.

Chapter 8

Protect Your Priorities from Too Much Screen Time

I didn't plan to write this chapter. But the more I researched procrastination, the more I realized I couldn't do justice to that topic without also covering the problems our phones have created. If I really wanted to help people stop procrastinating, I also needed to help them with too much screen time.

That's because too much time online is creating an unprecedented increase in procrastination around the world. Going online has become the number one avoidance activity—what most people do when they procrastinate instead of focusing on their goals. Some people have an addictive relationship with their smartphone and get anxious when it is even out of their sight. However, most people aren't addicted to their phones per se, but to the dopamine that is stimulated by the online platforms they access through their phones, computers, and tablets.

At the very least, addictions are bad habits that can place insurmountable obstacles in the way of your efforts to build good habits into your life. For many people, those bad habits have surged dramatically in the recent past. Food addictions are spiraling out of control, and more than 40 percent of adults in the U.S. are now considered to be obese. Obesity also affects a growing percentage of children. It's no wonder. The diets of Americans include more and more high-calorie junk food, and junk food manufacturers do extensive research to find the perfect combination of fat, sugar, and salt that will make you feel good and crave more. Alcohol consumption has also increased. Overdoses on strong feel-good drugs like fentanyl and other opioids have skyrocketed. Vaping with e-cigarettes has become much more common, especially among younger people. All of these are considered **substance addictions**.

In contrast, **behavioral addictions** are addictions to certain activities like gambling, shopping, and pornography. These have also exponentially increased over the past ten years. Corporate technology giants have discovered digital ways to hack into our brains, and the number of platforms available for potential online addictions seems endless. For example, addictions to internet platforms like social media and video games have exploded. Each platform is carefully designed by tech programmers to get and keep your attention for longer and longer periods of time.

What do all these food, drugs, and behavioral addictions have in common? Dopamine. This makes sense, because we live in a feel-good culture where immediate gratification, being happy, and having fun are some of our highest values. But **there's a dark side to dopamine**. Yes, it may lift you up, give you energy, and make you feel excited and happy in the moment. But too much dopamine overstimulates your brain. In an effort to restore its natural balance, your brain stops producing as much dopamine on its own. This means it takes more and more of the addictive substance or behavior to give you the same high. Plus, constantly overloading your brain with dopamine makes it difficult to feel happiness and joy from everyday activities like watching a sunset, listening to music, spending time with your family, and completing a challenging project. Addictions never make you feel happy or fulfilled in the long run. Instead, you're left feeling tired, annoyed, and craving your next mega-dose of dopamine to avoid being bored and feeling depleted and strung out.

All addictions, including internet addictions, cause changes in your brain. You become **obsessive** and can't stop thinking about your addiction. You become **compulsive** and can't stop doing whatever behavior gives you that dopamine high, despite increasingly negative consequences. Research shows your attention span gets shorter, your memory becomes impaired, and your mood takes a nosedive, which often leads to irritability and depression. In fact, **too much screen time results in the same changes in your brain as if you had been abusing substances like alcohol and cocaine.** The brain scans of people who are addicted to the internet and those who are addicted to alcohol and cocaine show similar impairments. Yikes!

Not only that, but by spending too much time online, you are knocking out the self-control center in your brain, your prefrontal cortex. This part of your brain is the adult in the room. As we covered earlier, it controls your impulses, provides you with willpower, and gives you the ability to anticipate future consequences so you can make long-term decisions that are in your best interests. Constantly flooding your brain with dopamine sidelines this Inner Adult part of your brain and allows the impulsive Inner Child of your limbic system to take over. You start living your life based on immediate gratification and what feels good now.

I got hooked on the internet during the COVID lockdown when everyone was advised to stay in their homes and not go anywhere unless it was absolutely necessary, like to get groceries. I don't have a television, so during that year-long period, my computer became my main connection to the outside world. I spent too much time online, and it affected my brain. I found it almost impossible to do the deep, critical thinking I needed to write this book because I couldn't follow an idea through to a logical conclusion. My memory was spotty. And I felt like I was on the verge of getting depressed.

I couldn't figure out why writing this second book was so much harder than writing my first one. It scared me because I didn't understand what was wrong with me. I was actually relieved to discover that my "cocaine brain" symptoms were the result of too much time online. Thank heavens I was eventually able to cut back, and my symptoms went away. If you're currently caught in a similar struggle, there's definitely hope for turning things around.

More and more people are waking up to the fact that they are online way too much. Surveys indicate that 63 percent of people would like to cut back on the amount of time they spend on their phones. That's a good thing, because the more time you spend online, the more likely you are to develop an internet addiction. And there is no immunity. Anyone can get hooked.

When smartphones became available, our vulnerability to getting addicted to our screens increased dramatically. That's when our access to addictive internet platforms became mobile. Now we carry our phones with us everywhere we go (even into the bathroom), which means we can get a hit of dopamine from our favorite online platforms 24/7. Anytime. Anywhere. Some people report they even check their phones during sex. I know. Surprising.

Help for addictions to substances like alcohol, drugs, and food is beyond the scope of this book. What I will do in this chapter is focus on internet addiction and share with you the things that helped me get a handle on my own overuse. I will give you some questions to ask yourself if you're not sure if your internet use is a problem. I will describe some activities you can try if you want to cut back on your screen time. And I will suggest additional resources for you to consider if you want to get help beyond what you can do on your own.

You might want to skip this chapter, especially if you don't think you have an addiction to your phone or to the internet. However, you also may be among the many people who underestimate how much time they spend online. Plus, the more you use the internet, the more likely it is that you'll get hooked. I encourage you to at least skim through this chapter so you will understand how it might help you or someone you care about who is struggling with too much time online.

What is the Goal Here?

If you were addicted to alcohol, you could stop drinking. If you were addicted to cigarettes, you could stop smoking. However, with internet addiction, abstinence is rarely an option. It's not practical to stop using the internet entirely. We live in a digital world that often requires us to go online. Besides, the internet is not all bad; it gives us access to invaluable information and resources. So for most people, the goal is not to avoid using the internet completely but to find a healthy balance between the time they spend in the real world and the time they spend online.

However, this balance can be deceptively difficult to achieve. We have become so addicted to our digital devices that our habitual overuse is often unconscious and automatic. We check, click, scroll, skim, surf, and "like" without even thinking about it. And the high-reward online platforms offer something for everyone: emailing, texting, shopping, gaming, gambling, pornography, and sexting, not to mention Facebooking, Instagramming, YouTubing, Snapchatting, tweeting, TikToking, Whatsapping, and more. People get so hooked on their screens and the dopamine they can access that they flunk out of school, lose their jobs, neglect their children, walk into street signs, fall off of cliffs, and contribute to the distracted driving that causes many tragic—and preventable—fatalities each year.

With such negative and catastrophic consequences as a constant possibility, it's even more important to create a healthy relationship with the screens you use to access the internet. Plus, our children grow up in an increasingly digital environment. My hope is that if you find some helpful techniques in this chapter for keeping a balance in your own life, you will teach those to your children.

First Things First

If you had a medical concern that was causing problems, you would probably first want to acknowledge the problems and then see your doctor to get a diagnosis. That way, you would know what you were dealing with and could get advice on what to do about it. I've found the same is true when you have a psychological or behavioral concern that is causing negative consequences in your life. Start by acknowledging that you're having problems and how those are affecting your life. This is an important and powerful first step because it frees you to start looking for solutions.

For example, do you know how much time you spend online on most days? Have you tried different techniques to cut back on your screen time but didn't succeed? If so, what techniques did you try? There's no judgment or blame associated with these types of questions. Your honesty with yourself is what's most important and what will help you move forward.

If you think you might be experiencing problems because of the time you spend online, or if you know for certain you need to cut back, either way, here's what surveys show over and over again. When asked to report the daily amount of time they spend online, the vast majority of people underestimate the amount of time they spend—by a lot. Because it's so easy to underestimate your online time, I encourage you to answer the following questions with a simple yes or no. These five questions are adapted from the Internet Addiction Test (IAT), which was developed by psychologist and internet addiction specialist Kimberly Young.

1. Do you stay online longer than you intended?
2. Do others in your life complain to you about the amount of time you spend online?
3. Do you often prefer to spend time online instead of spending time with others?
4. Do you lose sleep due to being online?
5. Do you find yourself saying "just a few more minutes" when online?

Here are some additional questions to answer, again with a simple yes or no.

6. Have you been dishonest with others about your internet use?
7. Have you felt guilty, ashamed, anxious, or depressed because of your online behavior?

8. Have you jeopardized close relationships or have you missed job, educational, or career opportunities because of too much screen time?

Your answers to all these questions will give you a good idea if overuse of the internet is a problem for you. I also suggest that you ask the people in your life how they see your internet use. Talk to your family and friends. Even young children can give you valuable feedback on how they feel about your screen time and how it is affecting them. These kinds of conversations can be a wake-up call and can give you more motivation to cut back. However, most people already know if they're spending too much time online because their lives start to unravel, usually in one or more of three areas: health, relationships, and productivity. Their health may suffer. Their relationships may start to deteriorate. Their work productivity may start to go down. And yet, their excessive screen time often continues and even escalates. This escalation is to be expected because as with all addictions, it takes more and more of the addictive behavior to get the same high.

Once you look at the symptoms and consequences of spending too many hours online, be careful about falling into a common pattern of feeling guilty. Instead, take that information and use it as motivation to find a solution.

Instead of feeling guilty, get smart about reducing your screen time.

Guilt puts the brakes on your efforts to change. It slows you down and drags you into low levels of emotional energy. As we have covered, guilt doesn't work to increase motivation and effort, so please let it go. Instead, get smart. Understand what's happening in your brain with dopamine when you spend too much time online and use that knowledge to develop a plan that will help you cut back.

When I first realized how bad my internet addiction had become, I felt like I must be a weak person, someone with very little willpower and self-discipline. But the more I read about online addictions, the more I understood how our human defenses pale against such an onslaught of dopamine overload that is intentionally created by the designers of the various internet platforms. One expert said it like this: "The problem isn't that people lack willpower; it's that there are a thousand people on the other side of the screen whose job it is to break down the self-regulation you have."

Once you know you are so unfairly outnumbered by tech programmers whose job it is to get and keep you hooked, you can start to get some distance and perspective on your unhealthy habits. These programmers and tech designers aren't deliberately out to hurt you. In fact, some of them want to do good in the world and want to protect their users from harm. But unfortunately, their business model is set up to reward employees and companies that hack into our dopamine channels in ways that keep us looking at our screens. It's all about the advertising money that goes back to them.

Here's how addictive these platforms and tech devices can be: many of the employees and owners of these tech companies won't let their own children use their products. Either that or they put strict limits on their use. That was the case with Steve Jobs and Bill Gates when their children were young. They knew upfront what the rest of us often have to learn the hard way.

Techniques for Reducing Screen Time

You may have already known that you need to cut back on your screen time. But if you answered the previous eight questions honestly, congratulate yourself for taking that important first step. It takes courage to examine your problems with an open mind. That courage, honesty, and open mindset will be strengths you can use if you decide to cut back.

Once I realized I had an internet addiction, I set out to learn everything I could. I read books and online material on screen-time addictions, and I experimented with lots of different strategies. Reducing my screen time was harder than I thought it would be, but once I did, my thinking and mood returned to normal. Thank heavens. But wow. That was frightening. Here are the techniques I found most helpful.

1. Increase Your Awareness

- **Learn more about internet addictions**

  Read books that describe internet addiction and why we are all so vulnerable. Learn how online platforms hack your brain to get and keep you hooked. A list of the books I found most helpful is included in the Recommended Reading section at the back of this book.

- **Increase your awareness about your patterns of overuse**

Notice when you go online but didn't plan to. Also notice when you stay online longer than you planned. What makes it harder to resist going online? What makes it harder to get off the internet once you're on it?

- **Write down your triggers**

Look for the triggers or cues that start your routine of overuse. Write down what you discover. Is it when you feel anxious, bored, or tired? Is it when someone pushes your buttons or makes you feel bad. Is it when you need to do something you don't want to do, so you procrastinate by going online? Is it simply a habit you do without thinking anytime you have a few minutes of free time? Write down the people, places, and things that start your addictive cycle.

- **Identify your problem platform(s)**

At the beginning of my "recovery" phase to cut back, I realized I couldn't completely avoid the internet. I needed to learn how to use the internet through moderation, not abstinence. What helped a lot was to realize there were only two platforms that were a problem for me: YouTube and online news sites. I didn't overuse email, texting, social media or other platforms. I only needed to focus on YouTube and the news. What about you? What platforms are a problem for you? Is it Facebook, Instagram or TikTok? Are you a gamer and can't control how long you play? Are you a shopaholic and can't resist searching for the next bargain? Zero in on exactly what platforms are hard for you to use in moderation.

2. Try Cutting Back

Now that you know what platforms cause problems for you, try cutting back. You can do this in several ways.

- Designate certain times of the day when you *can't* use the platforms. For example, I started by telling myself, "No news before noon."

- Schedule time during your day when you *can* use the platforms, and don't open them outside of your scheduled time. Later in the day is usually better than earlier.

- Decide in advance how long you will stay on a platform, then set a timer for that amount of time. This is helpful especially if you tend to lose track of time when you are on a particular platform. I don't recommend using your phone as your timer, for obvious reasons. Instead, I use a kitchen timer, which you can buy on Amazon for under $10.00. When your timer's alarm goes off, move away from your computer or put down your phone or device and start doing something else. Otherwise, you may be tempted to turn off your alarm and stay on the platform.

- Try changing *where* you access your problem platforms. For example, I tend to spend less time reading the news if I read it on my phone instead of my 23-inch computer monitor. Look for a location that will support cutting back.

- Make it harder to access your problem platforms. Remove the apps for your problem platforms from at least one of your devices— the one you most often use to access the platforms. Let's say one of your problem platforms is Netflix. If you can't log into Netflix automatically and have to go to their website and type in your credentials, this extra effort might help you become more aware of when you're starting to fall into your unhealthy habit. It can make you less likely to mindlessly go onto Netflix and get caught up in the dopamine it provides.

- Make a list of activities you can do besides going online. When the craving to open your problem platforms kicks in, you will need to find something else to focus on. Immediately. The longer you stay with the craving, the more likely you are to give into it. Make a list of things you can do besides going online *before* you need it. These substitute or replacement activities can make the difference between the success or failure of your efforts. Keep your list readily available. Don't keep your list in your phone if you think that accessing your list will make it too hard to resist opening your problem platforms. Here are some possibilities.
  - Take ten slow, deep breaths.
  - Walk. Around the room. Around your house or office. Around the block.
  - Write in your journal. Write down what you're thinking and feeling.
  - Remember WHY you don't want to open your problem platform. Write it down.
  - Call a friend or find someone to talk with. Distract yourself from your craving.

When you find yourself falling back into checking your phone or spending too much time online, simply ask yourself, "What else could I be doing?" If you have identified those other activities in advance, you have some alternatives.

- In addition to the activities you listed that you could do instead of going online, consider doing the Peace Process. If you can become aware of when you feel the urge to go online, of the instant you feel that craving, you can learn how to stop your impulsive habit. You can not only stop your automatic habit of acting on that impulse, but also release the feeling that may be causing your impulse and craving in the first place. Remember the four steps in the Peace Process: (1) pay attention (when you procrastinate), (2) find the feeling (in your body), (3) accept the feeling, and (4) act (by doing what you were stuck on). If you practice doing this enough times, you can release the underlying cause of your craving and eventually overcome your addictive behavior.

- Be accountable. At the very least, be accountable to yourself. At the end of the day, find a convenient way to record your progress on cutting back on your screen time. Write down exactly how much time you were on your problem platform(s). If you mainly access your problem platforms through your phone, you may be able to monitor your use by using a tracking app or the daily screen time function. You can also get weekly reports. For example, every Sunday morning my iPhone gives me a notification that says something like, "Your screen time was down last week by _____ percent for an average daily total of ____ minutes." Also consider being accountable to someone else, maybe a family member, friend, or coworker. This works especially well with someone who is also trying to cut back and reports daily or weekly progress to you. Quick emails or text messages to each other can be all it takes to help you both succeed.

3. Identify and Replace the Rewards from Your Problem Platforms.

Besides dopamine, identify the rewards you're getting from your problem platforms, which can be different with each platform. For instance, when I read the news, I often feel like the world is spinning out of control. When I feel a loss of control, I will try to get more information about why I feel that way, which keeps me reading more news, which makes me feel even more out of control. It's an endless loop. Plus, we live in scary times. As was the case with the Corona virus, what you don't know could kill you. So reading the news feels like a physical survival strategy. That's a pretty important reward.

We all want to feel in control. It's a natural instinct. There's nothing wrong with my desire to watch more and more news. I just had to realize that watching more news is never going to help me feel in control. I also had to acknowledge that I can't control what is happening in the outside world. At best, I can control what's happening in my own little world, in my own little corner of the globe. So now I focus on what I can control in my life. I find healthy ways to feel in control, like focusing on my writing and my health, staying on top of my other responsibilities, and meeting any deadlines ahead of time.

I keep an arm's distance from the news by limiting the amount of time I spend reading it to around twenty or thirty minutes a day. But I spend enough time to feel like I'm keeping up with current events and getting the health advisories, weather alerts, and other warnings that will help keep me safe. I don't want to stick my head in the sand and remain uninformed. Keeping abreast of what's going on is important for all of us. I just don't need to spend hours online every day in order to do that.

My other problem platform is YouTube. I notice that the YouTube videos I watch have different rewards. Some are entertaining. Some are educational. And some of the ones I get the most hooked on are inspiring. For example, one time I watched YouTube videos for three hours straight. I had no idea how much time had passed. I skipped my lunch and didn't even feel hungry. That time, I was watching old reruns of the singing competition, American Idol. Story after story of young people facing their fears and going for their dreams. Because those stories tap into the human spirit, they motivate and inspire me, and I notice I watch them when I need encouragement to keep reaching for my own dreams. If those young people can do it, I can do it.

My rewards for watching YouTube videos sometimes meet healthy needs in me. I don't want to completely stop watching them, and I can find other ways to meet the needs I get met through watching them. But I definitely need to cut back on the amount of time I spent so my behavior is more moderate and no longer out of control.

What are your rewards?
What about you? What are the rewards you get from your addictive

platforms? I suggest that you write down your problem platforms, the rewards you get from each one, and what you might do instead. Here are some rewards to look for, along with suggested replacements.

- **Social media**. Platforms like Facebook and Instagram can provide an instant community of "friends." Loneliness is another epidemic in this country and many other countries. Billions of people—young and old alike—get hooked on social media because it virtually connects them to others and makes them feel less lonely—in that moment—but only in a superficial sort of way. We all need human connections. The problem comes when we make the majority of those connections online instead of connecting with others in person. The research consistently shows that paradoxically, the more people use social media, the more lonely they feel. When you make more in-person connections in your life, you can diminish your need to spend too much time on social media sites.

Social media platforms also take advantage of our fear of missing out, often referred to as FOMO, along with our need for approval from others. The number of "likes" from others in response to our posts can make or break our day. We get hooked on fickle criteria such as likes, friends, and followers. It's no wonder people who spend more time on social media tend to have problems with anxiety, depression, self-criticism, and low self-esteem.

- **Computer games.** Online video games can also fulfill your need for connection with others. Some games provide instant "friendships" with others from around the world who are playing the same game. For those who are uncomfortable with in-person relationships, these games can be especially addictive. Their internet connections become their best friends.

Computer games can also provide challenges, competition with yourself and others, and a sense of accomplishment and mastery when users progress through the various levels in the game. All of those are basic human needs. Getting those needs met in the real world means developing practical skills and abilities that increase your competency and sense of self-worth. In contrast, only getting those needs met through online games proves to be a quick dopamine fix that is mainly a waste of time.

The key is to find and focus on healthy goals and challenges in your non-virtual, real life. Learn better organizational skills by decluttering your house or apartment, one drawer, one cabinet, one closet, or one room at a time. If you're a student, challenge yourself to get better grades. Start playing golf or tennis. Learn photography or how to play the guitar; you could watch YouTube videos, take an online class, or take lessons in person. The point is to find ways to learn, grow, and develop new skills in the real world.

Different platforms meet different needs. For example, online gambling may provide the risks, excitement, and suspense that's missing from your life. Online shopping may give you the adventure of looking for good deals and the pleasure of finding what you want at a rock-bottom price. If any of these are a problem for you, find healthy ways to get those needs met. I also suggest that you **look for healthy ways to replace the basic needs your online addictions are meeting as soon as you decide you want to cut back.**

Cal Newport, the author of *Digital Minimalism*, conducted an experiment to see what would happen when people took a break from the internet. The participants agreed to do a "digital declutter" for 30 days and not use apps and platforms that weren't absolutely necessary for their personal and professional needs. A journal entry from someone in the study read something like this:

> *I was surprised by how hard the first several days were. My addictive habits quickly became obvious. I would automatically reach for my phone while waiting in a line, when I was bored or needed a break, when I wanted to look up something, when I wanted to touch base with someone I'm close to. This went on all during the day and into the evening.*

Does any of that sound familiar? Probably. As this journal entry shows, we are deeply dependent on our phones for many reasons. No wonder we check them so often. But each time we check our phones, we risk opening the specific platforms that are addictive for us.

4. Follow This 8-Step Plan for Overcoming Your Addiction

If you really want to get serious about overcoming your internet addiction, I suggest you read a book called *Dopamine Nation* by Anna Lembke. She is the director of several addiction programs at Stanford University and a psychiatrist who works one-on-one with people who are addicted to various substances and behaviors. In her book, Lembke describes the eight-step protocol she uses to help her patients overcome their addictions. She used this same protocol to overcome her own compulsive behavior. I followed the steps myself, and they helped me break my addictive habits and get back on track with my life, starting when my internet addiction was at its worst. You may need additional help, but her protocol gives you specific steps to follow if you want to use a protocol that's proven to work.

What About Abstinence?

In order to overcome your internet addiction, at some point you will need to learn how to abstain and stop using your problem platforms. Or at least stop using them so much. Maybe you will have to stop using them altogether. Maybe you can learn to use them in moderation. But the bottom line is that cutting back on addictive platforms can be extremely difficult for some people. Please note this is not a suggestion that you give up the internet. Your only goal is to abstain from your problem platforms—not avoid going online altogether. You can still use the platforms and apps you don't overuse and the ones you use for your personal and professional needs.

I know a man who enjoyed online gambling for several years—until he lost a substantial amount of money. That's when he said, "Never again." For him, the risks weren't worth the rewards. I know other people who addictively played online video games every day, which resulted in lots of problems in their lives. However, once they abstained for a while, they were able to gain a sense of control over their gaming and eventually returned to recreational use.

Wherever you eventually land with your own addiction—whether it's total abstinence or occasional use—it helps if you first know what you're up against. You already know you are getting massive overdoses of dopamine from your screen time, which make you feel excited and happy. Plus, your addictive platforms usually help you meet other basic human needs and desires, like how social media can make you feel connected to others and less lonely in the moment, even if it's in a superficial sort of way. Overcoming your addiction means finding new ways to feel excited and happy, ways that don't involve going online.

Lembke and others have found that it takes about thirty days of abstinence in order for our brains to get back into balance. In order for our brains to start producing more of their own dopamine, which allows us to once again feel pleasure in everyday activities. This period of abstinence is sometimes called a **dopamine detox** or a **dopamine fast**. It is standard protocol in most inpatient drug addiction treatment programs; people start by abstaining for a month. Without that period of abstinence, it will be more difficult for you to think clearly and start to use your own healthy thinking to support your recovery efforts. But thirty days can be a long, *long* time to go without your addictive online platforms, especially if you spend hours online every day when you first start out.

Start Where You Are

When it comes to abstinence, **you start where you are**. If you can only resist picking up your phone to access your addictive platform for three minutes, then that's where you start. If you can only resist for one minute or even thirty seconds, then that's what you do. Stay busy. Use distraction. Earlier in this chapter, you made a list of things you could do besides going online, things like deep breathing, taking a short walk, or finding someone to talk to. The goal here is to resist your craving to go online for longer and longer periods of time. Experiment with different techniques that help you resist. In general, the longer you abstain, the easier it gets.

You will probably have a better shot at being successful if you practice your resistance first thing in the morning. Once you go online, once your brain gets that first taste of dopamine, it's harder to resist your craving to go online for the whole rest of the day. Plus, your willpower is strongest when you first wake up. It's like a muscle that gets weaker the longer you use it at any given time. However, if you practice strengthening your willpower muscle a little each day, then over time, it will eventually get stronger. Set up challenges for yourself where your goal is to resist temptation for longer than you did the day before. Record your progress. Add in plenty of rewards when you're able to resist for longer periods of time. But just to be clear, **it will be difficult to win any addiction battles by using willpower alone.**

Use Outer Game and Inner Game Techniques

You may need to use a combination of Outer Game and Inner Game techniques to succeed. You can start with Outer Game strategies since they are sometimes easier to put in place. The goal is to set up your environment in ways that make it easy to do the right thing and hard to do the wrong thing. In Chapter Four on Outsmarting Impulsiveness, we looked at things like: silence your phone, hide your phone, and block tempting sites. All these techniques can help.

If you're not sure you can stay off your phone, you might also choose a more radical approach by getting rid of your phone altogether. More people are getting rid of their smartphones—along with all the notifications and temptations they provide—by getting "dumb phones" instead. These are the earlier models of mobile phones that aren't connected to the internet. These people are tired of the constant interruptions from their notifications, and many want to avoid some of the struggle of resisting their cravings to go online.

A less extreme approach is to experiment with short fasts, like a week, a day, or even half a day. Some people have found that taking a 24-hour break from all their devices makes them feel so much better that they want to continue to cut back. As we covered in Chapter Four, if you're worried about missing an emergency call, use the Do Not Disturb settings on your phone to allow calls from certain contacts. Most Do Not Disturb functions will also override your block if you get two calls from the same person within three minutes, so you can let your emergency contacts know this in advance.

For suggestions on doing a 24-hour screen fast, as well as more techniques for restricting your phone usage, I suggest you read Catherine Price's book, *How to Break Up with Your Phone*. It can also be easier to cut back if you share your goals with someone else. Partners and married couples will sometimes decide to cut back together and support each other's efforts all along the way. Or find a friend, family member, or coworker who also wants to cut back. If nothing else, you can each use the other for support and accountability.

You can also use your phone itself as a form of support and feedback, a way to hold yourself accountable and measure your progress. Most smartphones have features that help you track your screen time. There are also lots of apps available for monitoring your screen time and helping you with time management in general. I'm not including in this book suggestions for specific apps. However, I encourage you to search on your own for those that will give you the feedback and accountability you need. Price's book also has lots of suggestions.

We also covered Inner Game strategies in Chapter Four like making a promise in advance and using self-talk to your advantage, including statements like, "Not now," and "Be strong right now and focus for five minutes." You're more likely to succeed if you use a combined approach: work to strengthen your willpower muscle a little each day, find healthy replacements for the needs you're getting met by your addiction, and figure out which Outer Game and Inner Game techniques are effective for you.

In the last chapter on healthy habits, I described additional techniques you can experiment with including: pre-commit to a date (when you will start your abstinence), use the 1% rule, and do the Peace Process. You can also shift your identity and start thinking of yourself as someone who knows you're being manipulated by the tech people who designed your addictive platforms. You're someone who is 100 percent committed to taking back control of your time. And you're someone who is more than smart enough to figure out how to develop a healthy relationship with your screens, a relationship where you enjoy the healthy ways you use your screens and avoid the unhealthy ways. You can turn these kinds of identity statements into affirmations, write them down, and repeat them (out loud) often. For example, say to yourself, "If I keep going and don't stop, I'm 100 percent certain I can learn to use the internet in healthy ways."

If you think you should wait and maybe detox later, do what Lembke does with her patients. Ask yourself these questions.

1. Do you want to still be dealing with this addiction in ten years?

2. What about five years?

3. Do you still want to be addicted a year from now?

These three questions can help you tap into the wisdom of your Future Self and find the strength to do a detox now. Because addictions are progressive, they get worse over time. Remind yourself that doing a detox later will be even harder.

If you think doing a 30-day detox is extreme, consider what happens in some other countries like China and South Korea. Internet addiction is such a problem there that young people sometimes go to internet "camps" where they aren't allowed access to any tech devices for several months at a time.

What I've Learned from Doing Dopamine Detoxes

I've now done six dopamine detoxes, each lasting anywhere from a week to a month, along with lots of shorter detoxes of only several days. I only abstained from my two problem platforms (YouTube and the news), but I can't tell you how much that helped. My fuzzy thinking cleared up after a few days. The longer I abstained, the better I was able to focus and concentrate. The cravings for these platforms went away after about a week, and I became off-the-charts productive, partly because I had so much more time to work on my goals. But here's the deal. As soon as I started going back to those platforms, my addiction returned almost immediately, and the cravings and addictive behaviors quickly ramped up to the levels where they were before, if not worse.

I realized I would always need to be on high alert for the possibility that I would fall right back into my old patterns if I didn't put some boundaries in place. I now use most of the techniques I described earlier and so far, so good. I still slip up sometimes. But I've managed to maintain a level of control over my screen time that prevents it from interfering with my goals. You can learn how to do the same. In most cases, you need to start by abstaining from dopamine overload and give your brain a chance to heal.

Just a heads up. I've found that it's much easier to stay on my dopamine fast if I stay busy with outside activities, especially when I first begin. That's why I often start my fasts on a day when my schedule is packed with activities that don't require using my devices, like grocery shopping, running errands, attending an event, or having lunch with a friend. Because the first few days of a fast are usually the hardest, keeping busy with these kinds of activities is one of the best ways to help yourself succeed. When you're tempted to give into your craving to go online, read through the list you made earlier of the things you could do instead. Distract yourself away from your craving by doing something else.

While you are fasting from your addictive internet platforms, it's also a good idea to find ways to increase your body's natural production of dopamine. Getting enough sleep, eating a healthy diet, exercising, and meditating can all boost dopamine levels and help your brain start to heal and function at its best. One of the biggest surprises that came from my internet fasts is just how often I go online when I needed an energy boost. A shot of dopamine from YouTube could quickly bring me out of an energy slump, so it's easier to be successful with my fasts if I think preventively and try to keep my energy levels up to begin with.

5. Get Outside Help

Remember, it's not your fault you got hooked on screen time. But it is your responsibility to change it. You may want to start by trying to cut back on your own by using some of the suggestions I just described. But if you give those a good-faith effort over a reasonable amount of time and they don't work, I suggest you ask for outside support. The possibilities for help are increasing and include online courses, one-on-one therapy, group therapy, and residential treatment programs. You also might want to check out a Twelve-Step program called Internet and Technology Addicts Anonymous (meetings are available online or by phone). I encourage you to search online, explore the available resources, and find the support that feels right for you. You could also look for a mental health professional who specializes in behavioral addictions who could help guide you through your choices.

6. Explore All Your Options.

So far, I've described several ways to overcome an internet addiction.

1. Increase your awareness (for instance, read books, observe your own behavior).

2. Use Outer Game techniques by changing your environment. Make it easy to do the right thing and hard to do the wrong thing. Examples include turn off notifications, hide your phone, and remove problem apps.

3. Replace unhealthy rewards with healthy rewards.

4. Use Inner Game techniques to change your behavior (long enough to establish new habits). These include discovering and challenging any limiting beliefs.

5. Get outside help. This can mean enlisting the support of family and friends, getting more information about internet addictions, and seeking professional help.

I have experimented with all the strategies I've described except for seeking outside professional help. But in a way I did get that help, because I did lots of reading and used the protocol for overcoming addictions that psychiatrist Anna Lembke described in her book, *Dopamine Nation*. By doing all these things, I found the strategies that worked for me and was able to control my screen time addiction well enough that it didn't interfere with my goals.

But to be completely honest, even after I found what worked for me, I still had a craving to go online and stay online way past any reasonable amount of time. And I had a fear that I would give in. That I would fall back into my old patterns if I didn't stay vigilant and guard against my craving to prevent it from stealing my time like it had so many times in the past. It was a healthy fear, but I didn't feel confident I wouldn't relapse.

Then something remarkable and completely unexpected happened. I watched a YouTube video by author and entrepreneur, Alex Becker, called "This Made Me Quit Alcohol Forever (You Will Too)." In this video, Becker describes how he stopped drinking by confronting his limiting beliefs about why he drank. Becker credits his success to having read *The Easy Way to Control Alcohol*, written by Allen Carr. As you may remember, Carr also wrote *The Easy Way to Stop Smoking*, which I described in the previous chapter on healthy habits, and which has helped millions of people. The key for Becker was realizing that alcohol provided no benefits in his life. None. In fact, alcohol took away from benefits like having fun, getting physically fit, and succeeding at his business. Once he could clearly see that alcohol was holding him back in life, then quitting drinking became an easy choice.

I don't drink, so that part of the video didn't apply to me. But as I listened to Becker, I realized I had two underlying limiting beliefs about my internet addiction. I believed that going online *relieved* my stress when actually, it was a SOURCE of stress. If I hadn't spent so much time online, I would have already done the things that stayed on my to-do list way too long and eventually stressed me out. I also mistakenly believed that spending lots of time online brought me pleasure, but in the long run, it brought me pain. It was a cheap thrill. It made me feel good in the moment but didn't add any value to my life. It stole the time I could spend doing things that were important and meaningful to me and made me feel like life was passing me by. Because in some ways, it was.

Wow. Those realizations changed the game. Almost immediately, my craving to go online vanished. I still had the *habit* of going online to deal with my boredom and stress, but my new awareness completely took away the physical craving and urge to go online. Without the craving to have to resist, it's been much easier to stay focused on my goals and enjoy healthy ways of feeling pleasure. And I'm not constantly afraid I'll fall back into my old ways of wasting time online like I used to be. My eyes are wide open. My awareness is too keen.

I'm sharing my experience with you in case you're still battling against your craving to spend too much time online. Look for any underlying limiting beliefs that may be causing you to think your excessive online time is a good thing. Then challenge those beliefs and keep reminding yourself that your beliefs were probably never true in the first place. This technique is different because it doesn't require willpower or self-discipline to work. If you don't believe your internet addiction adds value to your life but instead (in the long run) creates misery and pain, your newfound awareness can help remove your desire to spend too much time on your screens. In other words, when you eliminate the mental cause of the problem (your limiting beliefs), the problem will often go away. If you start to go online out of habit or out of FOMO, remind yourself of how grateful you are that your screen time is no longer controlling you. You are the one in control.

I was so inspired by Becker's video that I bought Carr's book, *The Easy Way to Control Alcohol,* and read it through, substituting my internet addiction for Carr's focus on alcohol. That further cemented my new belief that too much screen time was a complete waste of time. I later learned that Carr has published several other *EasyWay* books on topics like weight loss and quitting sugar and marijuana. He also has one called *Smart Phone Dumb Phone* which I plan to read next. Becker mentions in his video that he runs several multimillion-dollar businesses and is often asked how he stays so focused and motivated. He says if people would cut out alcohol, sugar, caffeine, and marijuana for 2 weeks, they would feel motivated, too. Interesting. Carr's books have helped millions of people around the world to do just that. They might be a good resource for you as well.

Just to recap, the bad news about addictions is that they hook us where we are the most vulnerable—through our DNA hardwiring for survival—which is to seek pleasure and avoid pain. The pleasure we receive from our addictions comes from massive overdoses of dopamine. The psychological and (sometimes) physical pain we avoid is often from current situations in our life and emotions that have gotten trapped in our bodies in the past. In the beginning, addictions make us feel oh-so good, and they effectively numb our bad feelings. They are a reliable source of pleasure and an instant anesthesia. But as addictions progress, they no longer provide pleasure. People compulsively go through their addictive routines just to avoid the pain of withdrawal and to numb out painful emotions they don't know how to manage. The good news is that once you understand what is happening in your brain when you become addicted, you can use that information to plan and support your own recovery.

Can everyone learn those lessons and recover from their addiction? Lembke has found that in almost every single case, the answer to that question is "Yes." People are doing it every day. Will you always be vulnerable to becoming addicted again? Again, the answer is "Yes." You may always tend to fall back into your addictive behavior if you don't stay vigilant and keep safeguards in place, especially when you're under extra stress. However, challenging any underlying limiting beliefs about your addiction can help protect you from relapsing. Is it worth it to take the time and effort to find techniques that work for you? Ask that question to the people who are in recovery, who have overcome their addictions and are now living happy and healthy lives. I, for one, can say from personal experience, the answer is an enthusiastic, wholehearted, and extremely grateful, "YES! Absolutely!"

As we covered earlier, one of the fastest ways to change a bad habit is to replace it with a good habit. We also looked at replacing the reward you get from a bad habit with something more constructive that will give you that same reward. But guess what? There's a replacement for your bad habit of too much screen time, something that is a constructive habit *and* that can make you feel even better. It's like a dopamine high on steroids. Only it's healthy for you. Plus, it will take you toward you goals instead of away from them. I will tell you all about it in the next chapter. Get ready to take your productivity to new heights. And get ready to feel a new level of amazing.

Chapter 8 Highlights

High five! Good for you for reading through this chapter. If you understand how addictions work, it's easier to use techniques that will help you protect your priorities from too much screen time. And that can make a world of difference in where your life goes from here.

1. Too much screen time is creating an explosion of procrastination around the world. Going online has become the number one avoidance activity— what most people do when they procrastinate instead of focusing on their goals.

2. The more time you spend online, the more likely you are to get addicted to the internet. Most people don't get addicted to their phones per se, but to the dopamine that is stimulated by the online platforms they access through their phones, computers, and other digital devices.

3. If you think you might have an internet addiction, or if you simply want to cut back on the amount of time you spend on your phone, there's definitely hope for turning things around by using the techniques described in this chapter.

Action Steps

Make a commitment to better control the time you spend online if that's a problem for you. Like me, you may find that taking control of your screen time will reduce your stress and make your life more enjoyable than you might expect.

1. Answer the eight questions that will let you know if too much screen time is a problem for you.

2. If you want to cut back on your screen time, experiment with the techniques described.

3. Keep experimenting until you establish habits that help you have healthy relationships with your phone and other digital devices.

Chapter 9

It's About Time

The digital age we live in has changed the tools and strategies we need to effectively manage our time. I've been teaching time management classes for years. We can still use many of the same strategies as before, but now we're up against a backdrop of nonstop tech distractions and interruptions.

Plus, our brains have changed because of the ways we use our tech devices. One of the biggest concerns I see is how our attention spans have gotten so much shorter. In the last chapter we looked at how to avoid too much screen time. In this chapter we will look at the broader issue of time management within the context of our digital environment. Be sure to read the latter parts of this chapter where I describe two time management strategies that can increase your attention span, concentration, and focus as well as skyrocket your productivity. But first let's explore how we've gotten where we are now.

When Steve Jobs introduced the first iPhone in 2007 he said, "Every once in a while, a revolutionary product comes along that changes everything." Boy, was he right.

The iPad came out in 2010, which further changed the digital landscape.

But it was during 2011-2012 when Americans experienced a digital shift equivalent to a seismic, nationwide earthquake. That's when the scales tipped, and more than half the people living in this country owned a smartphone. Our lives have never been the same.

Over time, our smartphones have gotten smarter, and they are now our personal assistants. They tell us what time it is, keep our calendars, send us reminders, and serve as our cameras, our maps and driving directions, and our connections to other people around the world. They provide access to every tidbit of information we might want; they're our dictionaries, our encyclopedias, and our 24/7 access to the news. They help us do our banking, pay our bills, and shop nonstop. With this one small device, we can check the weather, the stock market, and write a shopping list or an entire book. They're a virtual entertainment center, with instant access to music, television, movies, and a warehouse of online video games.

With all these useful and fun features on our phones, it's no surprise that our phones have also become our best friends. Studies show that 66 percent of us sleep with them. Many of us use them as an alarm clock to wake up in the morning. Even if we're not using them as an alarm, 89 percent of us check them within 10 minutes of the time we get up.

Our phones are our companions whenever we have to wait—in a line, for a doctor's appointment, for a stop light to turn green. And whenever we feel uncomfortable for even half a second, we can always reach for our phones, knowing they will provide a reliable source of distraction and an instant flood of dopamine that temporarily takes away even the slightest hint of discomfort. For many of us, they have become our drug of choice. We can use our phones to get a hit of feel-good dopamine anytime, anywhere.

The fact that our phones are wireless and can go with us anywhere has allowed them to become a convenient and almost irresistible intrusion into our lives. An intrusion that has had unforeseen consequences—both good and bad. But here are some alarming examples.

- Recent data indicates that the average American spends at least 10 hours a day on their screens. That includes their phones, computers, and other digital devices.

- Estimates vary, but they indicate that the average person checks their phone more than 300 times a day (one study found it was 344 times to be exact). If you account for eight hours of sleep in each 24-hour period, we check our phones an average of 21 times an hour throughout the day.

- Not surprisingly, our attention spans are shrinking. In 2000, the average attention span was 12 seconds. In 2015, our attention spans had shrunk by 25 percent, down to 8.25 seconds. Goldfish can focus on a task or object for 9 seconds. **That means our attention spans are now shorter than that of a goldfish!**

- Our phones and other devices constantly interrupt us with vibrations, pings, music, bells, chimes, whistles, whooshes, and whirs. These interruptions are expensive. If you are concentrating on a task and get interrupted—or interrupt yourself to check your phone or email—it takes 25 minutes after the interruption to get back to that same level of concentration. This lost time is called a **switch cost.** Because we check our phones and notifications so often, that means many of us never fully concentrate on anything throughout the whole day.

- Most long-term goals that provide high value require many hours of concentration and focus. With so many screen time interruptions, it becomes almost impossible to put in the time and concentration needed to complete these valuable goals. Because of this, businesses are losing billions of dollars.

- Not only are these interruptions and switch costs taking a toll on employee productivity, but it's also estimated that 71 percent of office workers abuse the internet during work hours by visiting social networking sites, shopping online, reading personal email, or visiting pornography, gaming, or gambling sites.

- College students sometimes fare even worse. A study done at Kent State University found that the more students used their cell phones, the more they fell behind their peers in academic performance, as measured by their cumulative GPA.

According to research conducted in 2023, the number of people who consider themselves addicted to their phones has now reached 57 percent. I think we can all agree that our screen time is out of control.

The recent avalanche of digital options is something we weren't prepared for and didn't see coming. There's no way we could have known that over the past few decades, tech programmers have been perfecting their strategies to hack into the ways our brains are hardwired for survival and use that to manipulate us into spending more time on our screens. We had no idea that each function, feature, and app on our phones was carefully researched and designed to be maximally addictive. But in fourteen short years, here we are. The question is what are we going to do about it? How can we take back control of our time and our lives?

Because here's the bottom line. Without a shift in our mindset and habits, many of us are likely to procrastinate on the things that are the most precious and important to us. Because of our hyped-up habits of checking and using our phones and other tech devices, we're likely to put off doing the things that are near and dear to our hearts. In short, our screen-time obsessions and compulsions may force us to give up what we say we want most.

You may be among the fortunate minority of people who don't check your phone hundreds of times throughout the day. But the *ways* we use our phones can also cause problems. That's because when most people are on their phones, they go into a "click daze" and quickly click-scroll-skim-swipe-repeat, constantly distracted and rarely staying on one screen for more than a minute. These frequent periods of focused distraction cause long-lasting changes in our brains and can make it more difficult to fully focus when we need to.

The rest of this chapter describes how to manage your time in our digital world, where many of us live every day in a state of information overload. Frazzled. Over-stimulated. Overwhelmed. And finding it more and more difficult to concentrate on any one thing for very long.

It's time for that to change, so keep reading.

Mindset Matters

The growing number of digital distractions means that managing our time and using it productively has gotten much harder. Not only that, but the pace of our world, and the speed at which our world changes have increased, causing many of us to feel like we're always driving in the fast lane, with no choice but to go faster and faster. Have you ever noticed yourself thinking or saying things like,

- There aren't enough hours in the day.
- I'm always behind.
- Gotta run.
- I'm overwhelmed by all the things I need to do.
- I feel like I'll never get caught up.
- No matter how much I get done, it's never enough.

These kinds of thoughts and statements can cause us to feel tense, anxious, frustrated, and afraid. It's hard *not* to feel this way when we live in a culture where there is always pressure to hurry and rush, where time seems scarce, and there's never enough of it. Our personal stories may also include time-pressure beliefs, which means many of us live with a **time scarcity mindset**, as if time is constantly in short supply. This chapter will give you the knowledge and skills to change those beliefs and instead, to live your life with a **time abundance mindset**, where time is plentiful and you don't have to rush all the time. You can still do what you want and need to do, only do it while you're feeling more relaxed.

As we have covered before, your thoughts and beliefs determine what you experience in the present and in the future. Although it may seem like a stretch, consider adopting a belief that says,

I have plenty of time to do what's important.

I encourage you to say that sentence out loud—right now—and see how that makes you feel. If you're like many people, you may feel some tension in your body or conflict in your mind if you don't believe that statement is true. However, if you continue to say that as an affirmation, and if you are open to the possibility that it might be true, you will likely start to feel your body and mind start to relax. You might even begin to feel a little more at peace. If you need some hope that this affirmation might be true for you, consider the fact that when you stop procrastinating, you will have tons of time you didn't have before. When you stop sabotaging your own efforts, you will instantly increase not only the amount of time, but also the amount of energy you have available to put toward achieving your goals.

Here's an example of how your beliefs about time and getting things done can determine what you experience. Not long ago I was in a grocery store when they were particularly busy. I only saw one employee working behind one of the counters, and when I placed my order I asked, "Are you the only one working right now?"

He replied, "Yes, for the next 45 minutes."

When I asked if that was stressful, his response surprised me. He said, "Not really. I used to work at a restaurant where we got really busy."

As I continued my grocery shopping, I kept thinking about the young man's reply, and I realized he managed to avoid the stress of what could have been an intensely stressful situation by using his thoughts. He didn't get caught up in the time pressure. He had learned ways to think about time-pressured situations in the past, and his thoughts determined his current experience. The lesson for all of us from this example is that especially when you're going through stressful experiences, **it pays to pay attention to your thoughts.**

Choosing to think empowering thoughts can help you stay calm and focused no matter what the circumstances. Being relaxed and calm can help you think clearly, rise above the stress of any situation, and take everything in stride. This is true in individual situations and in your life in general. If you experiment with getting out of the fast lane and use your thoughts to help you feel focused, grounded, and more relaxed, you may discover a better way to go through the time-pressured, extra busy experiences that inevitably come along. That's because

Calm is a superpower.

If your goal is to stay calm, relaxed, and grounded no matter what, it's easier to weather any storm. It's easier to consider your options, make better decisions, and act purposefully. Changing your thoughts and limiting beliefs about time and how much time is available can also open the door for you get more done in less time. It's paradoxical and seems almost too simplistic, but the more time you *think* you have, the more time you create and actually experience (as long as you're not using those thoughts to justify your procrastination). Thoughts become things. Your thoughts become your reality. Why not choose the thoughts that will lead to what you want?

And while you're at it, you might want to look at other areas of your life where you have a scarcity mindset. Maybe around money, loving relationships, or your health? Learn to notice when you are thinking thoughts of scarcity and change those into affirmations of abundance. Here are some examples:

- I have more than enough money to do what's important in my life.
- I am rich in relationships with people who love and support me.
- I enjoy establishing habits that lead to vibrant energy and abundant health.
- I'm grateful for the many blessings in my life.

Do these examples help you start to see the difference between scarcity and abundance mindsets? Here's a suggestion. Whenever you find yourself saying or thinking something that could contribute to scarcity in your life—stop. Let your awareness lead to a learning moment. Change what you're saying or thinking on the spot to something that is aligned with creating abundance and prosperity. And remember, you can always use gratitude to help create more abundance. As Willie Nelson said, "When I started counting my blessings, my whole life turned around." Feeling grateful for the abundance that's in your life right now and feeling grateful for the abundance that's not in your life—yet—is one of the best ways to create that abundance in the future.

Take 100% Responsibility for Your Time

One of the reasons time can seem so scare is because it's a nonrenewable resource. Once it's gone, you can't get it back. If you run out of money, you can always make more. If you lose love in your life, there is still hope. If you lose your health, it can often be regained. But when each minute of your life is gone, it's gone forever, never to return.

It's up to each of us to take responsibility for the limited amount of time we have on this planet and to use it in ways that make us feel happy and at peace. To live each day so that at the end of our lives, we have no regrets. Just like how Jim Rohn said, "You can't hire someone else to do your push-ups for you," no one else can take responsibility for your time but you.

We live in a culture of victimhood and blame. If something goes wrong or if we don't like something, there's a tendency to blame someone else or blame external circumstances for what we don't like or want. But by blaming outside circumstances, not only do you waste time, but you give away your power. If something outside of you is causing you to be unsuccessful or unhappy, that means you're dependent on that problem or external circumstance to change so you can succeed and your happiness can be restored. The goal here is to embrace your power to be successful and happy—*regardless* of the circumstances around you. Consider this quote by psychologist and author Albert Ellis,

> *The best years of your life are the ones in which you decide your problems are your own. You do not blame them on your mother, the economy, or the President. You realize that you control your own destiny.*

Once you take ownership of your experiences, you open the door to create the future you want. You embrace your own power to control your destiny. Other people and outside circumstances don't control you like they once did. You decide where you want to go, then do whatever it takes to get there.

Many people go through their whole lives feeling like victims of circumstances. They believe outside situations are causing their bad fortunes and bad feelings. It's not my intention to blame or shame people who truly are victims. For example, many marginalized groups of people truly are victims of systemic victimization like discrimination. Many of us have been victimized, and certainly most of us have felt like victims of circumstances at times. For instance, natural disasters can make all of us feel like victims. But taking responsibility for your circumstances means you own your **"response-ability."** You take ownership of your ability to *respond* to whatever happens. You may not be able to change the external circumstances, but you always have choices about how you respond to what happens. You can choose responses that leave you feeling less like a victim and instead feeling more empowered.

Some people go so far as to believe **everything that happens *to* you is happening *for* you.** This philosophy is based on an underlying belief that by choosing an empowering response to whatever happens, and by learning the lessons each experience can teach you, it's possible to turn what may initially look like bad fortune into good fortune. They believe every cloud has a silver lining, a hidden gift, or gifts. And one of those gifts is that you can use any "bad circumstance" to become stronger, wiser, and more skilled at responding to the next bad circumstance that will inevitably come along.

There's a quote by author Garrison Keillor that, "Nothing bad ever happens to writers; it's all material." I can't tell you how many times I've used that quote to see the gifts in what might initially look like bad circumstances. Like when I realized I was addicted to the internet. At first, I was shocked and thought it would make it harder for me to move forward in my life. And it did—for a while. But then I decided to write about my experiences of overcoming my addiction and to include all of that in this book. In the long run, I think my bad circumstance made this book more helpful to readers. At least I hope it did.

Here's a story that further illustrates my point. This is the story of a farmer whose horse ran away. Upon hearing the news, his neighbors came to visit. "Such bad luck," they said sympathetically.

"We'll see," the farmer replied.

The next morning the horse returned, bring with it three other wild horses. "How wonderful," the neighbors exclaimed.

"We'll see," replied the old man.

The following day, the farmer's son tried to ride one of the untamed horses, was thrown, and broke his leg. The neighbors again came to offer their sympathy for what they called his "misfortune."

"We'll see," answered the farmer.

The day after that, miliary officials came to the village to draft young men into the army. Because the son's leg was broken, they passed him by. The neighbors congratulated the farmer on how well things had turned out.

"We'll see," said the farmer.

The moral of this story is that you never know what gifts are embedded in what may look like bad circumstances. Consider adopting a belief that what happens to you is happening for you. Then choose an empowering response. If you respond with a "We'll see" attitude, you give yourself some time to look for the hidden gifts. And those gifts may eventually help change your destiny for the better. In other words, allow for the possibility that all your bad circumstances might contain gifts in disguise.

This same principle applies to your procrastination. Even though you may feel like a victim of your procrastination because of the amount of time you've wasted, it's always possible to find gifts in your experiences. For instance, your "bad circumstances" might make you even more determined to squeeze every ounce of productivity and enjoyment out of your time from now on.

Become a Student of Your Own Life

It's surprising how many circumstances can make me feel like a victim. Like one night of too little sleep. Being in a toxic relationship. Being in a job that's not healthy for me or not a good fit. All the scary things that are happening in our world like pandemics, extreme weather, an unstable economy, and political conflicts. There's no shortage of circumstances any of us could find to feel victimized.

One of the more useful lessons I've learned in my life is that when I feel like a victim, it's a sign I have one or more lessons I need to learn. And the sooner I learn those lessons, the sooner I can move out of a victim position and back into feeling more in control. The lesson is to **move from victim to student.**

211

Victim -> Student

Like most people, I feel powerless and out of control when I experience myself as a victim. But thankfully, I've learned those feelings are signals to think of myself as a student who needs to learn my lessons. The first step is to acknowledge that I feel like a victim. I also acknowledge any additional emotions I might be feeling—maybe betrayed, hurt, or angry. After that, I ask myself, **"What's the lesson I need to learn?"**

In any experience where I feel victimized, there are usually at least three lessons that can help me turn that experience into something that is empowering: (1) lessons that will help me get out of that particular situation (either leave the situation or change the situation to make it better), (2) lessons that will help prevent that situation from happening again in the future, and (3) lessons about how to get more skilled at learning my lessons faster. For example, if I don't sleep well one night, I immediately become curious and start looking for reasons I might have gotten a bad night's sleep. Then I look for things I can do differently the next night so I can get plenty of quality sleep. In other words, I become a student whose main mission is to learn the lessons embedded in my victim experience.

Many of the clients I counseled over the years came to me because they experienced some kind of trauma that made them feel like victims. In many cases, they truly were victims of circumstances. Some of them had at least partially healed from their trauma. But they were still having problems in their lives because they got stuck in their victim mindset and mentality. They still thought of themselves as victims. They hadn't learned the lessons that would help them move out of their identity as a victim so they could recover completely and move on with their lives. The moral of their stories is to keep looking for lessons that will help you fully recover and heal.

Besides having more lessons to learn, sometimes people who get stuck in a victim mindset have expressed their emotions around that trauma, which often has the added benefit of helping them develop insight and understanding into what happened. However, as we have seen, insight is often not enough for people to change their behavior. Insight and emotional expression may also not be enough to help people fully release their emotions, and they may still have an emotional residue of feelings that is trapped in their bodies, as I mentioned earlier. In other words, they have done what they could psychologically to heal the trauma, but there is still a chemical block of emotions in their bodies that needs to be released.

In these situations, using some type of mind-body technique to release this physical block can make the healing complete, as was the case with the Sandy Hook victims. If you have been procrastinating on a goal for years, consider using the Peace Process or some other mind-body technique in case your procrastination is due to a chemical block in your body.

Pay Attention to Your External and Internal Focus

Now that you know the advantages of taking 100 percent responsibility for your experiences, let's zero in on what that means when you take responsibility for how you spend your time. It's easy to feel like a victim of outside circumstances that so often interrupt your plans and require your time. Your child gets sick. Your work schedule changes. You discover a water leak under your kitchen sink. Your friend is going through a crisis and needs your support. Life happens. As we will discuss in more detail later in this chapter, you're probably doing well if you can stick to your time schedule and focus on what's important 80 percent of the time.

When those inevitable interruptions intrude on your plans, what matters most is how you respond to them. Do they completely throw you off track so you take forever to get back to your priorities? Or can you take them in stride and immediately return to what you had planned to do? When life interrupts their plans, people who are highly successful can quickly get back to focusing on their priorities. Those who are less successful struggle to get back to what's important and end up wasting a lot of time. This difference in the way successful and unsuccessful people respond is consistent with the age-old wisdom that

Where you focus your attention in the present moment creates your future.

Mahatma Gandhi said it like this,

The future depends on what you do today.

You may be thinking that this is common sense. Of course, what you focus on now determines what you experience in the future. Taken a little further, whatever you focus on expands. You create more of it.

And yet many people get stuck at this point. They think about what they want in the future. They set goals. They may even visualize what it will look like when they successfully complete their goals. But they don't *take action* on those goals. They don't DO whatever it would take to make those goals a reality. Or they talk about all the great things they plan to do but never ACT on those plans to make them happen. They trick themselves into feeling like they are working toward their goals when they're only thinking or talking about them. Or they feel like they are working on their goals when they're doing busywork instead.

I spent a lot of time thinking about writing this book. Some of that time was productive mental planning. But thinking about writing doesn't make it happen. At some point, I had to stop thinking about writing and just do it. I had to put in the hours of writing time, sitting at my computer typing words on a blank page in order to reach my goal. Can you see the difference?

This example illustrates how staying focused on what we want in each present moment can be tricky, because we have an **external focus** and an **internal focus.** Your external focus is usually obvious because it's when you use your external senses. What are you looking at? Are you listening to something in your environment? What are you touching and physically doing as you interact with your environment? When I write, I'm looking at my computer monitor. My fingers are typing on the keypad. My external focus is clear.

In contrast, your internal focus has to do with your inner environment, with the thoughts and self-talk that run through your head and take up your mental time. It's your internal dialog, that voice inside your head that comments on your life—all the time—with or without your awareness. Your internal focus is time spent that you can't physically see. But as Louise Hay said,

Your current self-talk is creating today and tomorrow, as well as the weeks, months, and years ahead.

It's estimated that around 60,000 thoughts go through our minds every day, and about 80 percent of them are negative. These thoughts include our internal dialog when we say things to ourselves like: *I don't feel good today. I wish I didn't have to go to work. Why is that person so annoying? Is my friend mad at me? My hair looks awful. Why can't I lose weight? I dread having to finish that project. I have to make more money! I'm tired. I'll never get everything done.* Without realizing it, these kinds of thoughts can become an endless stream of internal negativity. They are part of the Inner Game of fears and limiting beliefs that make up 80 percent of the reasons why we get stuck in our lives.

These kinds of negative thoughts can create insurmountable roadblocks to succeeding at our goals. The key is to become aware of the thoughts and take responsibility for changing them to something positive, or at least neutral. But our thoughts can be illusive, and it's sometimes hard to know what we're thinking. One way to become more aware of your thoughts is to notice what you're *doing*, like when you procrastinate or when you're tempted to procrastinate. See if you can identify the thoughts that are causing you to put something off. Another way is to identify your negative thoughts is to notice what you're *feeling*. If you're feeling scared and afraid, it's probably because you are thinking fearful thoughts. In contrast, if you are feeling motivated, strong, and determined to reach your goals, it's likely because of your confident, can-do thoughts, whether you're aware of them or not.

Challenge yourself to become more aware of the thoughts that are running through your head. Then ask yourself,

Is this thought helpful?

Is any given thought helpful and supportive of you and your goals? Is any given thought taking you toward your goals or further away from them? Does any given thought make you feel uplifted and empowered? Or does that thought make you feel anxious, overwhelmed, or defeated? When you discover thoughts that aren't helpful, experiment with changing them to positive affirmations using the techniques we have covered previously in this book. Techniques Seven, Eight, Twelve, and Thirteen in Chapter Five can be especially helpful.

I need to make a special note about using Techniques Seven and Eight in Chapter Five, the ones that describe how to work with your Inner Child when it sabotages your goals. Whether you think of this part of yourself as your Inner Child, or your subconscious mind, or simply a part of your brain, sometimes we need to listen to what it is saying, especially to things that it keeps repeating. You may have heard that recurring dreams keep repeating because they are trying to give you a message. The same can be true for recurring thoughts. In other words, **sometimes our recurring**

negative thoughts have an important message we need to hear. Maybe that message has to do with our health or safety. Or maybe it is trying to help us solve a problem in our lives. The message could be about anything.

For example, if you have a recurring negative thought like *You're so lazy you won't even walk around the block*, that thought may be telling you to pay attention to your health by exercising, even a little. If you have a negative thought that keeps saying *You're terrible at managing money*, it may be trying to help you start saving for a time in the future when you will need some extra cash. Look for any valuable messages that might be embedded in your negative thoughts before trying to change them or just make them go away. Then act on those messages and take care of whatever they may be instructing you to do.

Once you determine there's no value in your negative thoughts, sometimes you can simply ignore them and they will start to fade away on their own. To shorten the time this takes, you can also experiment with talking back to the negative thoughts, either out loud or just to yourself. For example, challenge the truth of those thoughts by saying things like, "I don't believe you. You're not even true." Or say things like, "You used to help me out, but now I've outgrown you. It's time for you to go away" or "You're not helping the situation. Please leave. Now." After you say things like this, then switch your thoughts into DOING something productive by saying things like, "Right now I'm going to open my laptop and finish that report." These suggestions are in addition to other techniques described in Chapter Five. Allowing your negative thoughts to run rampant can create a huge obstacle to your success.

Another internal obstacle for many people is that without realizing it, **they focus on what they don't want—not on what they want.** It's so easy to fall into this trap. You need more money, and you focus your internal time and attention on not having enough money. In various ways, your thoughts keep repeating *Not enough, not enough, not enough*. What you're doing is creating a future where you still don't have enough money. Or you want a special relationship, and you constantly think about being lonely and not having that special person in your life. When you focus your internal attention on your scarcity and lack, it brings more of the same into your future. I've heard it said that "Worrying is like praying for what you don't want." So many times, this is true.

And if all that is not enough, your mind can be filled with negativity, not only from your own thoughts, but also from your environment. If you watch much news, you get mega-doses of negativity. If you spend much time on social media, you're more likely to become anxious, self-conscious, and depressed. If you're around people who are stuck in their lives, people who are blamers or complainers, or people who always seem to be angry, their negativity can rub off on you. If you don't take care of your health, your body can become a constant source of stress and negativity that can make you feel bad and drag you down every single day. All this negativity can make it much harder to stay focused on your goals and get things done.

At times, we all need to deal with external and internal negativity and conflicts; it's part of life. But as we covered before, a good rule of thumb is to **live your life so at least 80 percent of the time, you're focused on influences that are positive and helpful.**

Be intentional about protecting yourself from negative influences in your external environment and instead, fill it with things that are positive. Here are some examples. Keep your house and your life organized and uncluttered. Spend time with people who are positive and upbeat, who support you in reaching your loftiest goals, and who are stretching to reach their own. Read biographies of people who defied all odds and achieved amazing feats. Watch motivating movies. Read self-help books that can teach you specific skills you need to master. Listen to music with inspiring lyrics and sing along with the words. (If singing makes you self-conscious, do this when you're alone, like when you're in your car.) Spend time in nature. Establish healthy habits around your diet, sleep, and exercise, habits that will give you lots of energy and help you feel good physically.

Also, work toward creating an internal environment that is 80 percent positive. Focus on thoughts of abundance instead of scarcity. Instead of thinking about what you don't have, be grateful for the things you do have. Instead of focusing on the obstacles you're facing, focus on solutions and ways to get around those obstacles. Think about the things you *can* do, not on what you *can't* do. When you feel victimized, ask yourself "What's the lesson I need to learn?" then look for the gifts that situation may have for you. Focus on your strengths, not your weaknesses. Focus on your courage, not your fear. Focus on the goals you want to achieve, along with the thoughts that will motivate you to ACT to achieve those goals.

As we covered earlier, once time is gone, it's gone forever. You can never get back the time you've wasted. However, by spending more of your current external and internal time focused on what you want, it's possible that **you can make up for lost time**. You can start to move toward your goals faster and easier. The rest of this chapter describes more tools and techniques on how to do that.

Finding Flow

One of the ways you can protect yourself from too much screen time is to replace it with something that is far better. That is more fun and more exciting. A higher high. And not only that, but something that helps you achieve your goals, not avoid them. Something you want to do because it has its own built-in motivations. Something you can look forward to when you wake up in the morning.

You may have heard of **peak performance**. It's often used to describe the experiences of athletes when they accomplish what seems not only improbable, but even impossible. It's also called being **"in the zone,"** where people can perform amazing feats with seemingly little effort. Like making an unbelievably long putt in golf. Miraculously snatching an overthrown pass out of the air to score a touchdown in football. Firing off a long shot in the final seconds of a basketball game, making the shot despite the pressure, and winning the game. But peak performance and being in the zone don't just pertain to sports. That zone is something all of us can find in our day-to-day lives once we know how to follow the steps to get there.

This superhuman ability for optimal performance has been studied extensively, starting with Mihaly Csikszentmihalyi, a Hungarian-American psychologist at the University of Chicago. Early in his career, Csikszentmihalyi became fascinated with how artists who were painters would forget everything else while they were working. When they finished their work of art, instead of enjoying it, they started a new painting. They weren't interested in the final product. What they wanted instead was the experience of being fully absorbed in their act of creation.

This observation sent Csikszentmihalyi on a mission to find out what causes people to feel happy and content. His research started with athletes and artists. Then he expanded his focus to include musicians, chess masters, and surgeons. By working with other researchers around the world, he was able to get interviews with more than 100,000 people and ask them to describe their optimal experiences, the times when they most enjoyed themselves and felt the happiest. They included men and women of all ages and from all walks of life. Many of these people described times when their work seemed to "flow out" of them with very little effort. Because of these common descriptions, Csikszentmihalyi decided to call this experience **flow**. Based on his research, he wrote a book called *Flow*, which became a bestseller.

You may remember times when you experienced this flow state. It's when you become completely absorbed in a task. Nothing else seems to matter. Time becomes distorted and seems to either speed up or slow down. The experience is so enjoyable that you would do it even when it's expensive, for the sheer sake of doing it. (For example, winter ski resorts thrive on people who go into flow while skiing down their slopes.)

You can spontaneously go into flow when you're intensely focused on an activity, and especially if you are trying to get better at it. It's more likely to happen when you challenge yourself to stretch past your comfort zone but not stretch so far that you get overwhelmed or can't succeed. You aim for that place that's in between too easy and too hard. You can also focus on a goal that's naturally easy for you but do it in ways that make it more challenging, like cleaning your house, only do it faster or more efficiently without letting it become stressful.

What are some other characteristics of flow? It's when what you're doing seems effortless and easy. You feel in control and unstoppable, and there's a euphoria that makes you want to keep going. You get a break from your normal thoughts and any sense of self-consciousness or self-criticism. I experience periods of flow when I'm singing or dancing. You may go into a flow state when you're working out, playing sports, listening to music, or concentrating intently on your job. It's when you're completely caught up in the moment. It's a unique feeling of ecstasy and magic. And it can provide a source of motivation for achieving even your most tedious and challenging goals. Here's why.

The Problem with Goal Setting

There's a problem with goal setting that few people talk about. It's that the happiness that comes from accomplishing your goals doesn't last. You spend your time and energy diligently focused on achieving your goals, but when you reach them you're not happy for long. A coworker once told me she thought if she could just afford to buy the sofa she wanted, she would be happy. Indefinitely. But then she said, "I was so disappointed because when I finally got the sofa, I was only happy for a few days." I've had that same experience when buying a new car. I'm so excited before I buy it and when I buy it. But within about three weeks the excitement is gone, and it seems like just another car. This happens even when we reach our most exciting goals. Then we have to look for another goal to pursue in a never-ending cycle where happiness is a moving target.

That's because our desires are endless. As soon as you achieve one goal, more goals pop up to take its place. This goes on throughout our lifetimes, which makes it important to come to peace with any aspects of goal setting you might find frustrating. It helps if you practice keeping an attitude of gratitude for all the things you have accomplished, as well as feeling grateful for those things you haven't yet achieved.

Another solution to this dilemma is to enjoy the *journey* of moving toward your goals. In other words, **find a way to enjoy the journey... AND the destination.** Learn ways to be happy as you are working on your goals and moving toward your destination of achievement. Dopamine can help you do this. But dopamine is short-lived and can only take you so far. There's another way to approach your goals that can make even your most dreaded goals something you enjoy working on, and that is to **focus on your goals when you're in a state of flow.**

Why does the flow state help you enjoy the journey toward reaching your goals? Because there are two types of motivation: **extrinsic motivation** and **intrinsic motivation**. With extrinsic motivation, your desire to succeed is controlled externally by things you want or don't want. You want to buy a sofa or car. You want a promotion at work. You want your house to be organized and not messy. You want to avoid a late fee so you pay your bills on time. This type of motivation doesn't last long.

In contrast, intrinsic motivation is when you do something because you love it, because you love the way it makes you feel. According to Csikszentmihalyi, **the highest intrinsic motivation is a state of flow**. Musicians lose themselves and their sense of time when they completely surrender to the moment. Surfers wait for hours to ride waves that provide a thrill like no other. Rock climbers and sky divers risk their lives in search of a high that feels better than anything else they've found.

The good news here is that once you learn how to go into the flow state, you can focus on goals you may not initially love to work on. You can tap into the internal motivation provided by flow to accomplish goals you might otherwise avoid and even dread. For example, I usually love to write. But writing this book required so much research that I started to dread it, which led to avoidance. Then I learned how to go into flow. Now, despite the research I continue to do, I love writing again because I first follow the steps that lead to flow. You can learn how to do the same thing with even the most humdrum tasks and chores.

Here's another example. I had a workman in my house for two days while he put in new flooring, and he spent much of that time in a flow state. He had been in the flooring business for about twelve years, so it could have been boring for him. But he focused on working faster and more efficiently, without losing any of the quality of his work. We talked about his process, and he told me he loved his job because of the high he could achieve by continually trying to get better at it. Yes, he got paid for his work, so there was extrinsic motivation. But his main motivation was intrinsic. He had learned how to keep his job challenging and enjoyable despite years of practice.

The Power that Fuels Flow

What makes the flow state so enjoyable? And why do people all over the world describe it in the same ways? Steven Kotler is a noted expert and author of several books on flow, including *The Rise of Superman*. According to Kotler, dozens of neurochemicals in our bodies create the experience we call flow, which is different from all other states of consciousness, including drug-induced altered states. That's because: (1) flow is always a positive experience and (2) flow enhances your performance, whatever you're doing. Researchers have discovered more than twenty neurotransmitters that contribute to the flow state. The top five-star performers are dopamine, norepinephrine, endorphins, anandamide, and serotonin.

Kotler says these natural biochemicals have an extraordinary ability to boost your mood and enhance your performance. Together, this potent cocktail can not only enhance your individual performance, but also the performance of people working in teams or groups. In addition, it creates the kind of social bonding that can make you feel like you're falling in love. For example, when combined, dopamine and norepinephrine can give you that energy rush, hyperactivity, loss of appetite, excitement, and the giddiness of romantic love. Who doesn't love the feeling of being in love? Besides the emotional high, these neurotransmitters also make our bodies and our minds faster, stronger, quicker, more focused, more alert, and more creative. No wonder so many people perform at their best during flow and often feel it's magical. Not only that, but people who experience flow states also report they are happier and more satisfied in their lives—in general.

Addictions to mood altering drugs are at all-time highs in this county.

Health issues are exploding, and death rates are soaring due to our relentless pursuit of the next high that will help us instantly avoid pain and feel more pleasure. In addition to that, promising you ways to enhance your performance has become a business worth billions, from energy drinks that rev you up, to vitamins that claim to help you focus, to the whole arena of performance-enhancing teachings and trainings. It's paradoxical, and heartbreaking, to realize that so much of what we seek outside ourselves to enhance our performance is available to us naturally and for free by learning how to use our inner resources in ways that produce flow.

Steps for Finding Flow

Are you ready to learn how to go into flow? The flow state can be illusive. Especially when you first start to experiment with intentionally going into flow, it can be difficult to create. You can't *make* it happen, and sometimes too much effort gets in the way. But you can make flow more likely to happen by following the three steps described below. The steps aren't hard. But just like learning how to dance, you need to practice them until they become automatic and you get better at going into flow when you want. With enough practice, you can learn how to reliably go into flow practically every time you try. Here's what to do.

Step 1: Choose a clear goal

To get started, identify a goal you want to achieve, something you already know how to do, but you want to get better at. For example, this could be getting better at a physical skill, like playing a sport. When I worked in a university athletics program, I saw how most of the athletes found flow during their practices and competitions. That's why they loved their sport and why they had gotten so good at it. They constantly challenged themselves to improve. You could also choose as your clear goal a mental skill like meditating or writing reports. Maybe you want to get better at a hobby or learn how to do mundane chores faster and easier. For example, see how fast you can pick up the clutter around your house and still stay relaxed. I call this technique **picking up speed without picking up stress**, and it can add challenge to almost any chore or routine activity. Also, choose a good time to focus on your goal. This is usually in the morning when your willpower and mental energy are at their peak. However, if you're a night owl and concentrate best in the evening, use these same steps to enter flow at a time when you think it will work best for you.

Step 2: Focus on immediate feedback

Next, when you focus on achieving your goal, figure out what will give you immediate feedback on what you need to do to improve. For instance, if you're playing soccer, how can you get better at kicking the ball so it goes where you want it to go? Focus in on how to improve your kicking skills and keep practicing. If you're trying to learn how to play tennis, maybe zero in on your backhand and keep practicing how to make it better.

As you stay focused on the feedback that tells you if you're getting better, push yourself out of your comfort zone of what's normal for you. Stretch beyond the level of skill you may have reached in the past. Your goal is to use the feedback from your efforts to help you get better. Use more effort. Try new approaches. Experiment with different techniques that may help you improve. Then see what happens. Use that feedback to keep stretching to develop a higher skill level.

Step 3: Find your optimal challenge/skill ratio

When your focus on your goal of getting better, there's an ideal ratio between the difficulty of the task—your **challenge**—and your ability to perform the task—which is your current level of **skill**. If you challenge yourself too much, you will get anxious and may feel overwhelmed and discouraged. If your challenge is too easy, you will probably get bored and stop paying attention. You want to find the place in between when a task is too hard and when it's too easy. In other words, the task is hard enough to make you stretch, but not so hard that you become indifferent or want to give up.

As it turns out, there's an **optimal challenge/skill ratio**. If you push yourself to perform a task at a level that's 4 percent above your current skill level, that ratio forces you to focus intently and give it your all. What's so cool is that if you keep practicing getting more skilled at your goal, if you keep striving for a 4 percent increase in your skill level day after day, here's what happens. You get into a state of rapid growth. Each day you stretch to get 4 percent better than the day before. After ten days you could increase your skill level by 40 percent. And after 100 days, you could get 400 percent better. This rapid growth is how professional athletes manage to keep breaking world records. They push themselves to get better every day, and eventually they may end up among the most highly skilled in the world.

These are the three basic steps that can help you get into flow. There are additional factors to consider, like eliminating all distractions and making

223

a 100 percent commitment to becoming a master at whatever skills you want to improve. If you're interested in learning more about how to go into flow, I've included recommended reading at the back of this book. And if you need an incentive to learn more, keep in mind that studies show that people who regularly used flow states to achieve their goals **increased their productivity by 500 percent.** They also **increased their learning speed by 490 percent**. Wow.

Tips and Techniques for Managing Your Time

Focusing on your goals while you're in a flow state is one of the best time management techniques I've ever even heard of. When you're in a state of flow, you can accomplish things in hours that might otherwise take you days, or even weeks. And your creativity is off the scale. Many of humanity's greatest advances have been accomplished when people were in a state of flow. Consider these examples. Einstein was in flow when he finally figured out the theory of relativity. Marie Curie did her research on radiation when she was in a state of flow, giving us the use of x-ray technology in medicine, among other benefits. Sam Altman and his team at OpenAI (Artificial Intelligence) were in flow when they coded chatGPT (Generative Pretrained Transformer), and who knows where that will lead? These flow breakthroughs have permanently changed the direction and speed of our forward progress. You can learn how to do the same thing in your own life.

However, you can't stay in a state of flow for more than several hours each day (probably four hours max) because it requires massive amounts of dopamine and other neurochemicals. In flow, you're so highly focused that after several hours, you get too tired to continue. It's not sustainable over long periods of time and you need other tools and techniques besides flow to help manage your time. There are tons of excellent strategies in other books. I include some of my favorite time management books in the Recommended Reading section at the back of this book. Also, the first book I wrote, *The Power of Life Lessons*, includes an entire chapter on some of the strategies my students, clients, and I have found most helpful.

In the following information, I describe additional techniques you can experiment with to make better use of your time. I suggest you pick one or two techniques to use now. If they work for you, use them long enough for them to become habits. Then come back to this chapter and pick a few more.

The Rearview Mirror Technique

Many of my clients have made quick improvements with their time management by first identifying how they waste time. This imagery technique can help you identify and eliminate the activities that waste your time, often because they are simply bad habits. Do you know what your biggest time waster is? Maybe television? Social media? Netflix? Write it down now. Also, what's the worst distraction you struggle with? Is it notifications on your phone? Saying "No" to others? Also write that down. Whatever is a problem at the time, you can use this imagery technique to help yourself stay focused and on track. I call it **the rearview mirror technique**, and here's how it works.

First, pick either a time waster or a distraction you want to eliminate. You can also choose a bad habit, addiction, or an avoidance activity you want to stop doing. For a long time, for me, that was watching too much online news. Next, pick a symbol that represents that time waster, distraction, bad habit, or addiction. The symbol I picked was a screen shot of an online news page. Finally, imagine that you're driving down the road in your car and you look in your rearview mirror. In the mirror, you see the symbol of whatever you want to let go of. You notice that it's getting smaller and smaller as you drive into your future, leaving your unwanted behavior behind.

Once I practiced this kind of imagery a couple of times, I was surprised by how effective it had become. If nothing else, it helps me get psychological distance from whatever is causing problems for me. It also makes me feel more detached from the problem I'm experiencing and more in control. This imagery only takes a few minutes. I encourage you to practice doing it until your time waster or distraction is no longer a problem.

Consider ROI

There is a term in the business world called **ROI** which stands for **return on investment**. It is used when you make decisions about financial investments and want to consider how much return you will get from the money you invest. As a simple example, if you plan to sell your house, consider how any improvements will affect the value of your house when it's time to sell. It makes sense to put money into improvements that will give you the best return on your investment and increase the sale value of your house the most.

This same technique applies to decisions you make about how you spend your time. When you decide on your priorities and what goals are most important to you, consider the value that achieving those goals will bring in your future. In this case, "future value" can be different for everyone. Maybe right now you want to spend your time on goals that will bring you lots of money in the future. Or maybe you want to focus on goals that will give you optimal health so you get to physically feel good in the future you're creating.

To determine your personal ROI for how you spend your time, answer the following question. Your answer can help you decide what to focus on during your flow time, especially when you consider what will help make your current situations better *and* what will make a big difference in your future. This powerful question comes from a book by business coach Brian Tracy called *Eat That Frog* which became an international best seller. Ask yourself,

> ## Which one project or activity, if I did it in an excellent and timely fashion, would have the greatest positive consequences in my work or personal life?

You can apply this question both to your big picture goals and to smaller goals you choose to focus on in each moment. But just a warning. If you take this technique to heart, you may become more uncomfortable when you waste countless hours every day watching television or going down the rabbit hole of too much screen time. And that's a good thing.

Use the Pareto Principle

This technique is an extension of the one I just described on ROI. You may have heard of the Pareto Principle. It's often called the 80/20 rule. This principle says you get 80 percent of the value from 20 percent of the work. For example, if you have a to-do list of ten items, you will get 80 percent of the value of all ten by completing the most important two items, or 20 percent of the entire list.

The Pareto Principle generally holds true in other situations as well. For instance, in any given group of people who are working together, 20 percent of the people will usually do 80 percent of the work. This principle can be frustrating when you're always among the 20 percent of what I call "worker bees." But it can also be helpful to know the division of labor among most work groups.

Many business coaches have learned that by focusing in on the small percentage of priority activities—sometimes even less than 20 percent—businesses can increase their growth and productivity by a disproportionate amount—sometimes more than 80 percent. That's why they often advise their clients to use the Pareto Principle. Gary Keller and Jay Papasan are business coaches whose book *The One Thing* became a best seller. When they applied the Pareto Principle to their own business, they decided to publish a book that described their business services as "the one thing" that would provide the greatest value to their clients, the greatest ROI. Because of that decision, Keller scheduled his morning hours so that time was entirely devoted to writing the book. He did all his other work-related business later in the workday.

My own experience has been almost identical. I decided that completing this book would provide the greatest future value for my own business. I focused on my writing during my morning golden hours and took care of other activities and responsibilities later in the day. The fact that you're reading this book right now is a testament to how effective this technique can be. I encourage you to experiment with using it in your own life.

Schedule It

Once you decide on the top 20 percent of your goals, and after you identify "the one thing" that has the greatest value, schedule time when you will focus on that goal and only that goal. Find a block of time that is at least two hours long when you can devote 100 percent of your attention to that one goal, even if that means getting up early in the morning. You will have a better shot of going into flow if you schedule your priority during the golden hours, first thing in the day. We covered this earlier in Chapter Four, and I still recommend that you at least try to train yourself to use those early morning hours on work toward an important goal, even if you normally concentrate better later in the day, and even if you need to go to bed earlier. To change your bedtime, turn off all your digital devices, including your television, two hours before you plan to go to sleep. The blue light from your screens interferes with your body's natural rhythms of getting to sleep and staying asleep. If early morning simply doesn't work for you, find another block of time and schedule that for your top priority.

Just a note here. We all have an **internal prime time**, when we focus and concentrate the best (We covered this in Chapter Four). Do what you can to use this prime time to focus on your most important goals. However, some goals require us to interact with others. We need to talk with others and use normal business hours to complete our goals. When that's the case with your priorities, you will also need to consider what's called **external prime time**, the time of day when you can connect with resources that will help you complete your goals.

Whenever you schedule your priority, make certain there are absolutely no distractions. None. Turn off your phone. Hide it. Put it in another room if you need to. Turn off all notifications on your computer. Enlist the help of others by asking that they not interrupt you during this time. This is your time to make magic happen in terms of how fast you accomplish your goals. Don't let interruptions stop you from doing that.

Once you take into account your internal prime time and the external prime time you may need, you're ready to schedule into your calendar all the activities your top priority will require. Write those times down in your calendar. Do this each evening when you know how much you've gotten done that day. If you need to change one of your top priority times, be sure to schedule another time to make it up so you don't shortchange the weekly amount of time you spend. When the time comes for you to work on your goal, show up ready to dial in. Challenge yourself to work with focus and intensity. Give it all you've got for that block of time. You may be surprised by how much more enjoyable your activity can become simply by not holding back and not getting interrupted while you're working on it.

And remember, unscheduled, open times are when you might be most likely to slip into an avoidance activity that can throw you off your schedule. I'm not suggesting you book yourself into time slots every hour of the day. Just be aware of when you might be vulnerable to falling into procrastination and schedule low energy-demand activities at that time if you need to. If you do schedule most of your time, cut yourself some slack when life's unexpected interruptions get in the way. A realistic goal is to stay on your schedule 80 percent of the time. Another rule of thumb is that it's not realistic to expect yourself to work on goals that require deep concentration for more than about five hours a day. Our brains aren't wired to go much longer than that.

Also, I've found that using the sport psychology imagery the night before makes it easy to remember and achieve my goals throughout the day. That's because all during the night, my subconscious mind already had a chance to practice being successful. And here's one final tip on scheduling. Author and life coach Jack Canfield swears by this and even calls it life changing. He calls it the **Rule of 5**, which is that every day, do five activities that will take you toward your top priority goal. These can be small, like sending a quick email or writing a to-do list for yourself. But they will give you lots of small "wins" each day and help you build motivation and momentum for achieving your ultimate priority. I agree with Canfield. This works.

Following a schedule can not only help ensure that you accomplish what you want. It can also bring you peace of mind. After one of my talks on procrastination, a retired gentleman came up to me and said, "During the week, I work on projects until 2:00 in the afternoon. After that, I can do anything I want." I sensed this was a happy and successful person, someone who worked hard and played hard. Just on first impression, he seemed confident and content with himself. I wish we could all be like that.

Create Morning and Evening Routines

This technique is an extension of the technique above on scheduling. I'm including it because what you focus on at the beginning and end of your day can make such a huge difference in your productivity and overall quality of life. Consider planning and scheduling these two times so you get the maximum benefits from where you focus your attention right after you wake up and right before you go to sleep.

Morning Routine

At the beginning of Chapter Seven on healthy habits, I told you Hal Elrod's story. Elrod was the young man who was hit by a drunk driver and was technically dead for six minutes. Because of his strong positive beliefs, he was eventually able to heal from his tragic accident, turn his life around, and reach even greater levels of success than he had before. But that wasn't the end of his story. After Elrod managed to create remarkable success a second time, the economy tanked. He lost his speaking and coaching business. He couldn't pay his bills. His positive beliefs couldn't save him, and he fell into a deep depression that seemed to have no end.

Elrod felt lost, with no hope on the horizon. In desperation, he started reading everything he could find about how to physically feel better. He asked everyone he could think of for suggestions that might help bring him out of his darkness and despair. Based on what he read and the advice of a friend, Elrod started running every morning. He didn't have the energy to run. He had no idea if it would help. But he did it anyway. And almost immediately, Elrod started feeling better. He started getting his energy back. His darkness faded away. And over time, his depression was gone.

Completely in awe of his own transformation, Elrod added more activities to what had become his morning routine of running. He experimented with activities that would help him get mentally and physically grounded and energized for the day and eventually developed a routine that took him about an hour. His routine included these six activities, which he called The Life S.A.V.E.R.S.

> **S**ilence (something like meditation – 5 minutes)
> **A**ffirmations (5 minutes)
> **V**isualization (5 minutes)
> **E**xercise (20 minutes)
> **R**eading (20 minutes)
> **S**cribing (maybe write in your journal – 5 minutes)

After experiencing the dramatic improvements his morning routine created in his own life, Elrod started sharing his story and his morning routine with others through a book he wrote called *The Miracle Morning*. The response was astounding. After reading his book, people from all over the world started developing their own morning routines and getting similar results, results that were life changing in so many positive ways. What began as one man's attempt to find a way out of his depression has grown into a worldwide movement because of that book. It has been translated into 37 languages, sold over three million copies, and is now practiced daily by people in more than 100 countries.

Here's my suggestion for you: read Elrod's book and create your own morning routine. Decide on a few activities that you think would help prepare you to have a good day, then experiment to see which ones work best. How you start your day makes a tremendous difference in how the rest of your day goes. By starting out focused and strong, you set the tone for what follows. You can use Elrod's six activities as examples of what you might want to include.

What I've found with my own morning routine is that I periodically need to change the activities so I don't get bored. It's possible to keep your routine interesting and energizing if you stay tuned to how each activity makes you feel. If an activity gets boring and goes stale, try switching to a different activity that gives you better results. Also, what you need from a morning routine can change over time. For example, if you've been sick, you may want all or most of your activities to focus on physical healing like yoga, gentle walking, and affirmations for health. If you've been particularly stressed, maybe you will want to spend more time on activities like meditation or journaling that will help you relax, stay calm, and get some distance from whatever has been stressing you out. Other examples of how to focus your morning routine include activities focused on improving your energy level, happiness, productivity, and financial prosperity.

The testimonials from people who started scheduling their own miracle morning activities are remarkable. People report things like doubling their income in a short time and quickly losing the weight they had been struggling to lose. Elrod explains that these results are because **the outside of our lives is a mirror reflection of the inside**. In other words, who you are as a person on the inside determines what your external life looks like, your external reality. When you grow intellectually, emotionally, mentally, and spiritually—as the Live S.A.V.E.R.S. support you in doing—your external reality will start to reflect that growth.

This principle of mirroring means that if you want to know what your beliefs are, just look at how you're currently living your life. It reflects your limiting and empowering beliefs, whether you're aware of them or not. Nine times out of ten, you can identify your beliefs by looking at how you're living your life right now. If you change your beliefs, your life can change accordingly.

That's why like many sages have shared, Elrod believes that **personal growth is the key to getting what you want in your life**. The people who enthusiastically endorse that principle and work hard on their personal growth during their morning routine quickly get hooked on doing it every morning because their results are so undeniable. Numerous studies have been done by interviewing billionaires, people who have managed to make billions through their own efforts. In almost every single case, they say they start their day early (around 5:30 a.m.) with a morning routine that includes activities for their health and personal growth, like exercise, meditation and reading. Even if your goal isn't to amass a fortune, the way you start your day can help you achieve whatever you want. Your morning routine can help you have the empowering beliefs, resourcefulness, and persistence to go after even your wildest dreams.

Evening Routine

As much as I value and enjoy my morning routine, I often think my evening routine is even more helpful. I like to wrap up my day feeling a sense of completion from the day's activities, so I pick up any clutter and put everything in its place. I want to wake up to a clean slate, ready for a fresh start. I also use visual reminders for tasks I need to complete the next day. If, for example, I need to return an item to a store the next day, I place the item by my front door. The same goes for any outgoing mail. Sometimes I will write myself a note to make sure I remember something like making a phone call to someone on their birthday. You can also send yourself reminders in your phone or schedule it in your calendar.

I like to end my day on a mental and emotional high note. While sitting on the edge of my bed (not laying down), I will think of at least one "win" I had during that day, something I did well, something I can feel thankful for and proud about. Then I will think through any "challenges" I experienced during the day, things I might not have handled the way I wanted. For example, maybe I got distracted and spent too much time online. After identifying a challenge, I will visualize a "happy ending" to that scenario. In other words, I will mentally "see" myself going through that same situation again, only this time, I handle it in ways that make me feel good about myself and make my response feel like a win. In this case, I visualize how I will avoid too much screen time in the future. Finally, I mentally say "Thank you" for the lessons that challenge is helping me learn. In other words, I find the silver lining to my challenge and end with a feeling of gratitude.

The last thing I do before laying down and falling asleep is visualize my ideal next day, how I ideally want to go through the next day, making sure I see, hear, and feel how I will successfully complete my goals—while I'm feeling calm and confident and enjoying each moment. For example, if I'm trying to establish a new habit, I imagine myself successfully doing that new habit, at the time in my schedule when I want to get it done. This visualization gives my subconscious mind the whole night to practice successfully completing my goal or habit and makes it easier to succeed.

Knowing what a good job my subconscious mind does with problem solving while I'm asleep, I often give it a problem or a question to work on during the night. For example, if I know I will be writing about a particular topic the next morning, I will often quickly skim through the material I'm likely to include right before I start my evening routine. Then I ask my subconscious mind to help me organize the material so I can write about it when I first get up. I'm floored by how many times I have an introductory paragraph in my mind as soon as I wake up, or at least a first sentence. Then all I have to do is write down what's in my head, and each time, the information I'm given and the way to say it seems almost perfect for what I need.

I love the fact that your subconscious mind can be practicing for your success all during the night, simply by what you focus on right before you go to sleep. That's also why it's so important that you not watch the news right before you go to bed. You don't want your mind rehashing that negativity all night long. I encourage you to experiment with both morning and evening routines. If you're like most people, you will probably be amazed at how much of a positive difference they can make in your life.

Use Monk Mode

The **monk mode** technique is a productivity hack that involves a short dopamine fast, similar to what we discussed in Chapter Eight. It's especially useful when you have a difficult project to complete or a deadline to meet in the near future. Here's how it works.

Set a challenge for yourself to abstain from all interruptions and distractions for a short time—maybe a few hours each day—or you can make it longer. Do this for however many days you need to complete your project. This means no screen time while you're focused on your project. Once you settle down to work and stop your mind from looking for constant distractions, monk mode will help you finish your work faster and easier. That's because as we saw earlier, each time you get distracted, it takes 25 minutes to bring your mind back to that same level of focus and concentration.

What I've described so far about using monk mode is the same as how you would normally schedule blocks of time on your calendar to work on your priorities. You want to avoid all distractions while you're focused on your goals. But monk mode takes this a step further. When you're in monk mode, you also **avoid all unnecessary distractions outside of your scheduled work times**. This means abstaining from all unnecessary screen time during the days and nights of your challenge. No unnecessary social media, texts, or emails. Minimal online news and television. Normal socializing with friends and family members is fine but wait on any extra socializing. Your goal is to temporarily eliminate many of the ways you normally get dopamine during your challenge. Also, as much as you can, avoid anything that's stressful until your challenge is over.

Without your screens to keep you occupied and distracted, you will have more time. You'll also get bored and will end up getting something productive done, almost in spite of yourself. Not only that, but as your dopamine craving increases, you can channel that craving into becoming even more productive, both with your priority project and with other activities on your to-do lists. Your increase in productivity will help you feel good about yourself and will start to build momentum for you to become more productive in general. In other words, **monk mode is a great way to make your boredom and dopamine cravings work in your favor.**

Some people try monk mode but feel too deprived. Or they set their challenge for too long and end up burning out. Remember, this is a meant to be a short-term challenge, probably no longer that a day or two. Or you can try it for several days, like on a weekend, especially when you're using this technique for the first time. You may need to start with challenges of no more than a few days then gradually extend those to last longer.

I encourage you to experiment with this technique because like with all challenges, there are lots of benefits. You prove to yourself that you can safely leave your comfort zone and nothing bad happens. You force yourself to stretch past your previous ability level and prove you're capable of doing better. You start to feel more self-confident and begin to see yourself as someone who can produce at a higher level, and your core identity starts to shift to a new normal. Your momentum increases. You may even start to build a habit of constant self-improvement, challenging yourself on a regular basis to stretch and grow into more of your potential. You won't know how monk mode might benefit you unless you experiment with it and find out.

I'm doing a monk mode challenge right now, as I write about monk mode. Not knowing what's going on in the news makes me anxious, but I have people who've promised to tell me if anything happens that I need to know about. Plus, I love realizing that when my challenge is over in a few days, I will have made lots of progress on my priority, which is finishing this book. I can always catch up on the news, and when I do, I'll be even more grateful I took this time out. I encourage you to try it.

Additional Strategies

Here are some additional tips to help you use your time more productively.

- **Beware of doomscrolling**
  I don't know anyone who feels positive and uplifted after watching

the news. But almost all of us subject ourselves to negative news daily, scared of what we will miss if we don't. We constantly scroll or surf through news sites, especially when the news is bad. We get hyper-focused on the content and can get hooked on the activity of scrolling. Not only can doomscrolling make you feel anxious, depressed, and afraid for the future, it can also disrupt your sleep, cause you to overeat, steal your motivation, and make it harder to do things you usually enjoy.

If you've fallen into the bad habit of doomscrolling and want to change that, start by becoming aware of when you're doing it. Use techniques previously described for breaking bad habits and building good ones. Avoid social media and other sites that focus on the darkness and negativity in the world. At the very least, set time limits for how long you will read or watch the news and use a timer to help you stop when your time's up.

- **Avoid Revenge Procrastination**

Do you ever stay up late at night to have "me" time, knowing you need to go to bed and get some sleep? This is sometimes called **revenge procrastination** or **revenge bedtime procrastination**, and it's more common than you might think. Lots of people put off going to bed in order to do things they didn't have time to do during the day, like watch their favorite television show, play video games, or catch up on social media. This form of procrastination can become a habit of staying up late night after night, even though you know you will feel exhausted the next day.

While out shopping, I ran into a friend I hadn't seen in a while, Stephanie. When I mentioned I was writing a book on procrastination, at first Stephanie told me she didn't procrastinate, that she had a strict schedule and stuck to it. I knew she had three children and worked long hours, so I took her at her word. But after I shared my struggles with spending too much time watching the news and YouTube videos, Stephanie seemed eager to tell me her problem was social media. She said, "I work all day, finally get the kids to bed, then I get in bed, planning to spend only a few minutes catching up on Facebook before I go to sleep. But I can spend two or three hours and not even know how much time has passed. I'm so tired the next day, but I keep doing it."

It can be easier to break this bad habit if you know what's causing it. Revenge procrastination is often the result of too little free time in your schedule. If that's the case, I suggest you change your schedule by setting boundaries on other activities and responsibilities, creating some unstructured time for yourself, even if it's just 30 minutes a day. That will make you feel more in control and will lessen any feelings of resentment or feeling like you "deserve" to stay up late because of all the things you've gotten done during the day. Also, revenge procrastination can be a symptom of burnout. Ask yourself if you might be burned out and if your answer is "Yes," look for more long-term solutions that will re-kindle your energy and create a healthy balance in your life. At the very least, schedule a realistic time to go to sleep every night and take small steps toward making it a constant routine. Your body will thank you.

- **Constantly Evaluate Your Progress**
You need feedback from your efforts to know if you're making progress on managing your time. Decide on what kind of feedback you want to monitor and evaluate your progress each evening. For example, if one of your primary goals is to simply stick to your schedule throughout the day, use that to evaluate how well you're doing. Maybe you stuck to your schedule 50 percent of the time. Or maybe you stayed on track 75 percent of the time. If your goal is to complete a certain amount of work during your scheduled times, use the amount of work you completed as your measure of progress.

As an author, I sometimes struggle to write a certain number of words or pages during a given time frame. Some content takes longer to write than other types, especially if I'm not familiar with it. In cases like that, instead of setting goals on the amount of content I want to write, I set what I call **time goals**. If I simply stay focused on writing for a certain amount of time, regardless of the number of words I write, I see that as success and get to count it as a win. Decide what you will measure to help you evaluate your progress. Figure out what works to help you reach your goals, then do more of whatever that is.

Remember the Compound Effect

You may have heard the time management advice to work smarter, not harder. The **compound effect** is a perfect example of working smarter. It's when you make small, smart changes to your behavior that have huge benefits over time. These little changes can make surprisingly big differences down the road.

Let's say you decide to eat fruit instead of a sugary dessert after dinner. By reducing your calories by a small amount every day, you will end up losing weight. No counting calories. No long, sweaty workouts at the gym. Making that one change to your diet may not be that big a deal, but over several years, you could end up being at a healthier weight, feeling better about your body, and feeling better about yourself. The benefits of your choices grow over time.

The compound effect is similar to saving money. Every time you put money in a bank account, your account gets bigger. Every time you invest in your health, your health increases. Every time you invest in self-improvement, the quality of your life gets better. Over time, you end up with remarkable results. The opposite is also true. Every time you take money out of your bank account, your account gets smaller. Every time you make bad choices about your health, your health declines. The results of your choices add up, and over time they either work for you or against you. The key is to remember the power of the compound effect and stick with your healthy choices for long enough to see positive results.

And not only that, but because of compounding, the positive results of your actions grow even more. If you have a bank account with a 5 percent interest rate, your money increases by that amount every day. On the second day after you invest your money, it increases by 5 percent. On the third day, it increases by 5 percent more than it was the day before. This goes on for weeks and months and years—however long you have the account. Over time, compounding creates enormous growth. You end up with much more money than what you invested. You get back more than you put in.

The same is true for other smart decisions to change your behavior. Maybe by losing weight, you have more energy to give to your relationships, and your relationships improve. Maybe your weight loss helps you be more positive and focused at work, and you end up getting a promotion or a raise. You never know how many positive results might come from one small, smart change. The key is to stick with your change until the results become obvious and start to give you motivation and momentum.

One of my coaching clients, Bob, struggled with procrastination, which had been a problem for him since he was a child. Bob's parents criticized him often, which made him feel like he wasn't good enough. He responded to their criticism by trying to be perfect. But because doing anything perfectly is almost impossible, he waited to even begin. Bob had good insight. He understood his perfectionism was the reason he procrastinated. But as is often the case, his insight wasn't enough to help him change his behavior.

Bob was a good father, and he raised his son, Jason, by using praise instead of criticism. Jason grew into a high schooler who felt capable of doing whatever he wanted in life. He would complete his school assignments right away, even if they weren't due for several weeks. He felt strong and empowered because he took charge of each assignment and had plenty of time to do his best work. Over time, the results of Jason's efforts paid off even more. Each success added to his bank account of self-confidence and made him feel more competent and assured that he would succeed with future assignments. In contrast, each time Bob procrastinated, it was like taking money out of his bank account of self-confidence, and he felt even worse about himself and his ability to succeed.

Which approach do you take? Are you more like Bob? Or are you more like Jason? Decide you want to be like Jason. Every step you take toward using your time wisely makes a difference in how you perceive yourself, your core identity. Every action you take toward overcoming your procrastination affects your bank account of self-confidence and your belief that *I'm good enough*. By experimenting with the time management techniques in this chapter and by using the ones that are effective, you can start to make the compound effect work in your favor.

Use the "Yes or No" Technique

I saved this technique for last because some people use it as a last resort to change their behavior. It provides a way to monitor your progress that forces you to increase your awareness of what you're doing moment by moment. You do that by constantly asking and answering this question: **"Am I focused on my goals right now? Yes or no?"** If the answer is no, write down what you're doing instead. Carry a pen and small notebook around and record your answers in that notebook. To avoid unnecessary temptations, don't use your phone for this. You can also jot down any other information that might help you see patterns in your behavior, like *when* you got off track and any other circumstances that contributed to your lack of focus (maybe you were tired or hungry).

One of the biggest challenges any of us face when trying to change our behavior is the fact that so much of what we do every day is unconscious.

According to biologist Bruce Lipton, because of our brain's software, we live 95 percent of our lives on autopilot. To keep us from having to make millions of decisions each day, our subconscious brain forms habits from the things we do repeatedly. We don't have to think about our habits, which frees our brains to focus on what's important in any given moment.

Want to brush your teeth? That's an unconscious habit. What about making your bed? It's probably unconscious. Drive to work? Likely you're on autopilot. If you want to change, you need to stop living automatically and do things differently. Change requires you to become more conscious and aware so you can live intentionally and on purpose. Using the "Yes or No" technique and writing down when you misuse your time is one of the fastest ways to increase your awareness and gives you some of the best chances to change.

Many people use a modified version of this technique to become more aware of their eating habits by keeping a food diary of everything they eat. Others use it to get a handle on their spending habits by writing down every penny they spend. I'm suggesting it here to help you become more aware of how you spend your time and to eventually take more control. The goal is to spend more time focused on completing your goals and less time on busy work, unimportant activities, and other time wasters.

However, you can't stay focused on your goals every minute of the day. You have other responsibilities and needs for other activities like eating, sleeping, socializing, relaxing, and having fun. But these other responsibilities and activities can support you in reaching your goals. They provide a healthy balance for you to have the time and ability to succeed at your top priorities. When you ask yourself the "Yes or No" question, answer with a "Yes" if you are doing something that supports your ability to work on your goals. Just be careful not to fudge and answer "Yes" when you're procrastinating or wasting time instead.

Once you learn how valuable this technique can be, consider using it—not as a last resort—but as the first strategy you use to change other behaviors. Want to stop being so sarcastic? Write down every time you say something snippy or sarcastic to someone else. Want to get more physically fit? Put yourself on an exercise schedule, then write down all the times you say "No" to working out. This technique provides invaluable, in-the-moment feedback, which is why it works so well. Just ask the many people who have used it and finally gotten the results they wanted.

Choose Healthy Dopamine Activities

This technique is different and one you probably won't find among other tips for managing your time. But it has the potential to radically improve your productivity, your life, and how much you enjoy your life. That's because it looks at which activities you use to reward your brain with dopamine. We know that dopamine is the primary motivator and reward for all behavior. It helps keep us alive. Without dopamine, we wouldn't have much motivation to meet even our most basic needs for things like food and shelter. When your dopamine level is low, you may feel tired, bored, apathetic, and even depressed. But as we have seen, flooding your brain with massive doses of dopamine makes you crave even more and makes it impossible to find pleasure in everyday activities. Overdoses of dopamine can also lead to agitation, obsessions, compulsions, and addictions. The key is to find healthy dopamine activities that help you maintain an optimal balance of this chemical in your brain. In other words,

The overall quality and enjoyment of your life depends on what activities you use to get dopamine rewards.

To live a successful and fulfilling life, it's essential to spend your time in healthy ways and in ways that provide the right balance of dopamine. Without enough dopamine, you will often default to the quickest ways to get higher levels of dopamine, like television, junk food, and the internet. But too much of these higher dopamine activities wipes out the healthy balance in your pleasure centers, and you will start to search for other activities that will further increase dopamine release.

You may find that you get a dopamine high from making money, but because that high makes you crave more, making money can turn into an addiction. You may go from occasionally using recreational drugs to regularly using prescription drugs. Celebrities sometimes go from the intoxicating levels of dopamine that fame and fortune provide to more massive dopamine activities like illicit drugs and sex. The same pattern can happen with people who are riding the waves of dopamine from their power positions, like certain politicians and some members of the ultra-wealthy. They keep looking for bigger thrills and higher highs. These kinds of destructive dopamine activities can destroy your whole life.

It's also important to look at how often you engage in high-dopamine activities. Too much alcohol on New Year's Eve or during a Super Bowl party is one thing. Getting drunk every weekend is something entirely different. Occasionally playing video games for a few hours as a reward for your hard work may be okay for you. Playing video games for hours every day is destructive. Keeping up with your friends through social media can be healthy and enjoyable. Too much time on social media is a time waster and can make you feel anxious and depressed. It's all about balance and moderation. It's all about time and the amount of time you spend doing healthy and unhealthy activities.

Remember, anything that makes you feel good is releasing dopamine. This includes all your unhealthy habits, the ones you wish would just go away. Once you understand that dopamine rewards are underneath all the activities you choose to spend your time on—the healthy and the unhealthy ones—it's easier to start spending more time in activities that are healthy. Here's how. Take the next five minutes to make two lists. On one list, **write down your unhealthy dopamine activities,** the ones that drown your brain in too much dopamine. These include eating sugar and junk food, using substances (like caffeine, alcohol, nicotine, and marijuana), and activities like too much television and screen time.

On the second list, **write down your healthy dopamine activities**, the ones that slowly drip moderate amounts of dopamine and help keep your brain's pleasure centers happy and balanced. These include enjoying a healthy meal, being productive and getting things done, learning new skills, exercising, attending sporting events, listening to music, any of the arts (singing, dancing, writing, painting), cooking, reading, gardening, and meditating. The overall time management goal here is to spend more time doing the healthy dopamine activities and less time doing the unhealthy ones.

Look at the Value You Get from Your High Dopamine Activities

There's something else we haven't explored yet, and that's the value of the activities that flood your brain with dopamine. Some high dopamine activities also provide high value, like flow. The creativity and productivity of flow is like nothing else. Going to a live music concert can be a high dopamine activity, one that is also extremely entertaining and can make memories that last a lifetime. Being productive, getting a lot done, and crossing things off your to-do list can also make your dopamine levels surge, for good reasons. But some of the activities you use to get a flood of dopamine are low-value activities. They may make you feel good in the moment, but they don't provide much value in your life. An example of a low-value dopamine activity is caffeine. Like sugar, it temporarily lifts you up but then drops you down where your energy levels are lower than they were to begin with. That's because substances like caffeine and sugar drain the dopamine out of you and inevitably lead to an energy crash.

I encourage you to examine the list of unhealthy dopamine activities you made, the things you do to get a dopamine rush but that aren't healthy for you. Go through your list and put a check mark next to the ones that don't provide much value other than immediate gratification. As you look at the marked activities on your list, ask yourself, **"Which of these unhealthy, low-value dopamine activities would I consider giving up?"** If you decide to get serious about letting any of them go, also think of healthy dopamine activities you might use to replace them. For example, you could experiment with giving up caffeine and replacing it with exercise.

More and more people are quitting caffeine habits they may have had for years and are finding they sleep better, are less anxious, and have more energy. To their surprise, they are also more productive than they ever would have imagined. If you want to see their testimonials, check out the growing number of videos that are being posted on YouTube. The point is to start looking at your unhealthy dopamine activities from a new perspective. Ask yourself if it's time to replace them with something healthy that still gives you a dopamine rush but also adds value to your life.

Here's another suggestion. Become more aware of when you have too little dopamine in your brain. Watch for things like boredom, complacency, junk food cravings, and urges to check your phone. If you have overstimulated your brain with too much dopamine (like with too much screen time)—when you cut back on that overstimulation—you may feel tired, sad, and unmotivated, and you may find that your brain is foggy and that it's hard to think. Also notice when you have too much dopamine, like when you've got a buzz from alcohol or you're in a TikTok daze. You may feel energized in those moments, but they are short-lived and an energy crash is coming. Either extreme can make you vulnerable to procrastination. Procrastination itself is usually an unhealthy, high dopamine activity. Because it's a habit and something you do again and again, you know it's triggering a dopamine reward. Putting things off or running late often gives you energy by releasing dopamine, along with adrenaline and other stress hormones.

Also, learn how to maintain a general awareness of the dopamine balance in your brain. This awareness can help you choose to spend more of your time on activities that give you optimal amounts of dopamine. Remember, the overall quality and enjoyment of your life depends on how well you choose. In order to live a happy and fulfilled life, spend the majority of your time doing healthy, high-value activities that release a moderate amount of dopamine. Not too little and not too much.

There's one more time management technique I want to suggest. I describe it in the next section on your Inner Witness, and I may have saved the best for last. That's because many highly successful people find that it's their favorite—their best and most enjoyable strategy for managing their time, day after day after day. Keep reading to see if you might be among them.

Discovering Your Inner Witness

Throughout this book, we've seen how awareness is the first step to change. If you want to change your thoughts, first become aware of them. If you decide to change your behavior, increase your awareness of what your behavior is now. Most of the activities and action steps I've suggested include increasing your awareness.

When you keep increasing your awareness, it's like exercising a muscle, and your awareness muscle will get stronger. You'll get better at self-awareness and will start to discover what is sometimes called your **Inner Witness**. This is a level of awareness that's like having a little bird sitting on your shoulder, and this little bird is observing what you're thinking and doing. It's not judging your thoughts and behaviors as good or bad. It's not trying to change anything. It's just noticing and observing what's happening in each present moment, in the here and now. The little bird is simply witnessing "what is" from a detached, on-your-shoulder distance. This means you can watch what your doing—while you're doing it.

Enjoying a Positive Addiction

When I'm in a Witness Position, my mind feels relaxed, my body feels light, and when I move, it feels like I'm floating. Whatever I'm doing feels almost effortless. I love it. In fact, taking a step back and observing yourself can be so enjoyable that it's been referred to as a positive addiction. However, unlike other addictions, there are no negative consequences. Only more and more benefits when you get to enjoy going through your day focusing on the things that are important to you, staying productive, and being rewarded with levels of dopamine that are just right—not too little and not too much. In his book *Eat that Frog*, Brian Tracy described it like this:

> *Here is one of the most important of the so-called secrets of success. You can actually develop a "positive addiction" to endorphins (and dopamine) and to the feeling of enhanced clarity, confidence, and competence that they trigger. When you develop this addiction, you will, at an unconscious level, begin to organize your life in such a way that you are continually starting and completing ever more important tasks and projects. You will actually become addicted, in a very positive sense, to success and contribution.*

> *One of the keys to your living a wonderful life, having a successful career, and feeling terrific about yourself is to develop the habit of starting and finishing important jobs. When you do, this behavior will take on a power of its own and you'll find it easier to complete important tasks than not to complete them.*

Tracy has had an exceptionally productive career. He has written over 70 books, coached businesses around the world, and spoken to more than five million people. And from what he's described, he's done most of this while enjoying the high of being in a Witness position. Now that's something to strive for.

The Witness Technique is similar to a technique called **mindfulness**. It's a type of meditation that began in the East with Buddhist teachings and has now become a mainstream wellness practice in America. It's even being taught in elementary schools. Becoming a witness to your own thoughts and actions is exactly what happens when you practice mindfulness. And the research is clear. This calm, detached observer position leads to a level of awareness that can give you immense power. The power to not only feel phenomenal, but also make clear choices and take strategic actions that will benefit you in the moment and in the future.

And do you know what else? It's sustainable. You can stay in an Inner Witness position all day long if you want. That's because it triggers moderate levels of dopamine and other feel-good brain chemicals. You're not overloading your brain and creating imbalances in your pleasure centers. In contrast, as mentioned earlier in this chapter, you can only stay in a flow state for a few hours at a time because it requires massive amounts of dopamine and other neurochemicals. In flow, you're so highly focused that after several hours, you get too tired to continue. It's not sustainable over long periods of time.

But here's the deal. Why not use both? When you learn how to go into flow *and* learn how to use the Inner Witness level of awareness, you can become unstoppable. Each has its own benefits and advantages. These are probably two of the most valuable time management techniques you'll ever run across. The good news is that they're both free. Their only cost is the time and effort of learning how to tap into them, then using them enough to see positive results.

Here's just one example of the benefits of using the Inner Witness technique. Years ago, Timothy Gallwey, a tennis coach and consultant, wrote a classic bestselling book called *The Inner Game of Tennis*. In his book, Gallwey describes how he taught people how to play tennis. He did this— not by teaching them the physical skills of the game—but by helping them get in touch with their Inner Witness, the part of their mind that observed their behavior and the thoughts that either criticized or praised them for what they did. Gallwey's students made rapid and dramatic progress, much more so than if he had used traditional techniques for teaching tennis skills.

Gallwey wrote several more books on the inner game, including *The Inner Game of Work* and *The Inner Game of Stress*, as well as inner game books on music, skiing, and golf. More inner game books from other authors followed on topics like baseball, basketball, and chess. The popularity of these books clearly showed that people understood how important the mental game can be, both on and off the court.

Here's another way your Inner Witness awareness can be helpful. Use it to overcome your addictions, including any addiction you might have to your phone. A study was done with a group of people who wanted to stop smoking. Some of the smokers used a standard stop-smoking program recommended by the American Lung Association. Another group was trained in mindfulness and practiced traditional meditation. The people who used mindfulness quit at twice the rate and relapsed far less often than those who followed the standard program. The ones who successfully quit learned how to simply observe their cravings to smoke and relax into them, not trying to change anything. By doing this, they were able to "ride out" their cravings without giving into the urge to smoke.

Here's why mindfulness works with addictions. Right before you start into any addictive habit, something sets off your craving. That trigger or cue can be a thought, a feeling, or a physical urge. Your triggers can be either conscious or unconscious, but they predictably lead to the beginning of your addictive habit. When you're practicing mindfulness or the Inner Witness technique, you simply notice your craving and triggers. You don't try to change them or make them go away. You simply observe your craving—along with the thoughts, feelings, and urges that may have created it. As you continue to witness your craving without judgment, it can start to diminish and can eventually go away on its own.

This is exactly what happens when you do the Peace Process. Only with the Peace Process, you find the physical place in your body where you feel the feeling or craving and stay focused on that part of your body until the craving is completely gone. As you might imagine, these techniques have the potential to completely turn your life around, then keep you headed in the right direction.

How to Strengthen Your Awareness Muscle

With so many benefits and potential uses for the Inner Witness technique, you may want to practice strengthening your awareness muscle. Here's my best suggestion: meditate. Some people automatically want to avoid meditation if they think it means a particular practice, like sitting still for a long time. But as described below, meditation can take many different forms. I encourage you to choose a form that is a good fit for you and spend some time meditating on a regular basis, even if it's five minutes a day. Or three minutes. Or even one minute. Every second you practice meditation is training your mind to focus longer, concentrate deeper, and start to reap some of the long list of benefits of meditation that have been shown through research. These include better physical and mental health (including reduced anxiety and depression); less stress; increased attention span and concentration; reduced memory loss; increased patience, tolerance, and kindness; and improved creativity and problem solving. That's an impressive list. Mindfulness—and practicing the Inner Witness technique—can also result in these beneficial results.

Here's a simple way to meditate. Watch your thoughts as if they are clouds in the sky. They come and they go. Don't get attached or involved with the content of the thoughts. Simply observe them in your mind. There's nothing good or bad about the thoughts. They're not right or wrong. You just notice your thoughts and let them go on their way. You can do this anytime, anywhere. If you have difficulty observing your thoughts, start by writing down what you are thinking. You can quickly make the shift from writing down your thoughts to observing them in your mind, as you are thinking them. At that point, imagine that your thoughts are clouds that drift in and drift out of your awareness.

With more **traditional meditation**, sit in a comfortable position with your eyes open or closed. Meditation is simply focusing on one thing for as long as you can. For instance, you can focus on a visual object like a candle flame. You can focus on a sound like the word "peace" by silently repeating that word every time you inhale. Or you can focus on something kinesthetic, a feeling in your body, which could be the movement of your breathing, your inhale and exhale.

Sometimes it's easier to keep your one-pointed focus if you close your eyes. Then concentrate on staying aware of whatever you've chosen to focus on. What you will notice is that immediately, all kinds of thoughts pop into your head. This is completely normal and to be expected. Just ignore the thoughts and return to your visual object, sound, or feeling. That's it. That's all there is to it. You just keep ignoring your thoughts and returning to your one-pointed focus.

As you do this, you may begin to feel relaxed, calm, and at peace. After your finish your meditation, you can learn how to extend these calm, peaceful feelings into whatever else you do. In other words, experiment with carrying these peaceful feelings with you into other parts of your life. This will make it easier to stay in an Inner Witness level of awareness throughout your day. Ah. So enjoyable.

Some people resist even the thought of meditating because it seems like it would be too boring. These people may intuitively know that traditional meditation wouldn't be a good fit for them. Fortunately, they often do well with something called **movement meditation**. You can learn the same focus and concentration skills when you're doing some kind of repetitive motion like walking or running. For example, silently say "peace" to yourself each time you take a step. Whatever repetitive activity you choose, find a way to keep your focus on one thing and let go of the thoughts that intrude on your concentration. Just make sure you pay enough attention to your surroundings that you keep yourself safe. There are many other types of meditation, including **guided meditation**, which is available for free on YouTube. I encourage you to look around and find something that works for you.

Many people get addicted to food, substances, or behaviors because they are afraid of their own thoughts. I ran across a fascinating study that showed just how far people will go to avoid whatever they may be thinking. During this experiment at the University of Virginia, people were asked to sit by themselves in a room for 6 to 15 minutes. They had nothing to do. However, if they wanted, the participants could give themselves mild electrical shocks. Surprisingly, many of the people chose to shock themselves rather than be alone with their thoughts.

As a counselor, I've seen again and again how many people also avoid their own feelings. They were taught to fear their feelings as children, so why wouldn't they still be afraid? However, avoiding your feelings can create a lifetime of misery. You spend your time constantly running away from emotions that are too scary to feel, which keeps you stuck and afraid. Meditation, mindfulness, and the Inner Witness technique can help you heal this bad habit. The people who stopped smoking using the Inner Witness technique not only overcame their cravings and addiction. They also learned how to stop being afraid of their own thoughts and feelings, which meant they could take back the power their thoughts and feelings had held over them in other areas of their lives as well. You can learn how to do the same thing.

Spending some time strengthening your awareness muscle is more than worth it. Just ask the people who learned how to play the inner game, the smokers who quit, and the billionaires who meditate daily.

Here's More Good News

Do you want to hear more good news? **We're hardwired to feel bliss—most of the time**. That's right. Candace Pert was an internationally recognized neuroscientist and pharmacologist whose research contributed to what is today called mind-body medicine. Pert was the person who discovered that emotions are actually biochemical modules that are found throughout the brain and body. After making this discovery, she concluded that we are meant to live in states of bliss. We just need to nurture our mind-body connections and allow them to provide us with an ongoing, natural high. Meditation and an Inner Witness approach can provide that nurturance and help us feel good from the inside out, without needing an external reason to be happy. Pert tells all about this in her book,

Molecules of Emotions. Based on her research, Pert also concluded that our minds and bodies are so integrated and so closely connected that we can think ourselves into being healthy, just like we can think ourselves into being sick.

Pert's assertions make sense. We already know that usually, our thoughts create our emotions. Most of the time, what you think determines what you feel. Negative thoughts and emotions cause stress, and stress causes as much as 90 percent of illness and disease. By observing our thoughts and carefully choosing what we want to think, we can start to keep our thoughts positive and feel good as a result. Not only feel good, but impact our bodies in ways that also make us healthy and happy.

I'm not talking about ignoring negative thoughts that might have some value for you. Or ignoring negative situations in your life that you need to deal with. I'm also not referring to fake happiness and plastic smiles that can cause you to lose touch with yourself. I'm saying that if you do the inner work to learn how to observe your thoughts—then CHOOSE to let go of any negative thoughts that don't serve you—you can learn how to be happy a lot of the time. Besides letting go of negative thoughts, you can also learn how to deliberately focus on positive thoughts. Thoughts of gratitude can take you to happiness in an instant. Thinking of what you *can* do instead of what you *can't* do will help keep you positive. Seeing the good in yourself and others is a surefire way to help yourself feel happy and offer support to the people around you.

Choosing a growth mindset and thinking positive thoughts is also one of the greatest tools you have available to overcome procrastination. No matter where you are right now, there's always the possibility you can turn things around. If you're still procrastinating and living in partial darkness, the light may be just around the next corner. Don't stop. Keep going. You now have all the knowledge and strategies you need to stop procrastinating and start living the life you were meant to live. The power is within you.

Chapter 9 Highlights

Learning to make the most of your time can be a lifelong process, but one that has tremendous rewards. Even small changes can make big differences in your productivity, your happiness, and your sense of fulfillment. But it's important to cut yourself lots of slack when your efforts to improve your time management skills don't result right away in the changes you want.

That's because as neurobiologist Bruce Lipton says, approximately 95 percent of what we do has become unconscious habit. It takes effort to make the unconscious become conscious, then change the new behavior into something you prefer over your old habit. Set a goal to regularly stretch past your comfort zone. Start small then build up to bigger steps. Hang in there. Stick with it. The changes you make to use your time in better ways will repay you for years to come. Here are the highlights from this chapter.

1. Many people are hooked on their phones. And no wonder. Each function, feature, and app was carefully researched and designed to be maximally addictive. But unless we cut back on our phone use, many of us will procrastinate and be forced to give up our most important goals and dreams.

2. In our fast-paced world, it's easy to feel like time is scarce. Instead of living with a **time scarcity mindset**, you can learn how to live with a **time abundance mindset**, which allows you to believe that *I have plenty of time to do what's important.*

3. When you take 100 percent responsibility for your time, you are no longer held back by blaming outside circumstances for your bad fortune or bad feelings. Yes, bad things will still happen, but you can own your **response-ability** to respond to what happens in ways that leave you feeling more empowered.

4. There is so much darkness and negativity in the world. This makes it even more important that you live your live so **at least 80 percent of the time, you're focused on internal and external influences that are positive and helpful.**

5. The overall quality and enjoyment of your life depend on what activities you use to get dopamine rewards. The goal is to spend most of your time doing things that provide moderate amounts of dopamine—not too little and not too much.

6. You can learn how to develop a **positive addiction to getting important things done**. The dopamine and endorphins that come from being productive make you naturally want to keep going. Over time, it will become easier to complete important tasks than not to complete them.

Action Steps

1. Inevitably, there are times when we all feel like victims in life. Victims of circumstances, of natural disasters, of other people, and of our own actions. When this happens, there's always at least one lesson to learn—maybe to leave the situation, change it, or prevent it from happening again. Whenever you feel victimized, **move from victim to student** and ask yourself, **"What's the lesson I need to learn?"**

2. The **flow state** is what you may have heard called peak performance or being "in the zone." Just like athletes, we can all learn how to reach this natural, superhuman state where things are effortless and you feel unstoppable. Experiment with the three steps for finding flow then use flow to achieve your most difficult goals.

3. More than 20 time management techniques are described in this chapter. Techniques like the compound effect, the rearview mirror technique, monk mode, and how to avoid doomscrolling and revenge procrastination. Pick one or two techniques. If they work, use them until they become habits. Then come back to this chapter and pick a few more.

4. Interviews with billionaires indicate that most have a morning routine that includes things like exercise, reading, and meditation. Follow the suggestions in this chapter for creating your own morning routine. There's a worldwide movement of more than three million people in over 100 countries who say they've used a morning routine to get incredibly positive, life-changing results.

Chapter 10

You Were Born to Shine

Congratulations! You made it to the last chapter. You stayed the course, hung in there, and read through the material that will help you finally stop procrastinating. Good for you. You deserve not only a pat on the back, but lots of rewards for your efforts. It's time to celebrate.

It's time to recognize your accomplishments and give yourself the praise you deserve. Allowing yourself to feel pride and satisfaction increases your self-confidence and makes you feel stronger, more prepared, and more likely to succeed when you take on the next challenging goal. Giving yourself a reward provides more acknowledgement of your success and can help you feel an even greater sense of self-respect for your strengths and who you are as a person.

You are a "do-er." Someone who gets on the playing field of life and plays the game all out. Someone willing to get some scrapes, cuts, and bruises when you take uncomfortable action on your goals because you know that you will heal quickly and end up ahead for having taken the risks. Someone willing to go through the fear and frustration that is part of any challenging goals—the ones that scare you and excite you at the same time. You know it will be more than worth your time and effort, along with the failures and mistakes you might experience along the way. You start to take your energy back, which means you are taking back your power. You start to love and validate yourself more, which means you aren't as dependent on others to provide that love and validation for you.

And while you're celebrating, be sure to thank yourself for being curious, willing to learn, willing to investigate yourself and invest in yourself, willing to be honest, admitting you want to change and need to change, admitting you've been holding back. Celebrating that you have and are sometimes taking uncomfortable action to change your future for the better. Yes. There's a lot to celebrate and be grateful for.

If you've done the activities in this book, and you're now finally overcoming your procrastination, you have taken a leap forward that is probably much greater than you realize. When you find success doing something that has repeatedly held you back in the past, it's so empowering. Because underneath that accomplishment, you have done the inner work that proves the incredibly powerful fact that

You are enough.

Acknowledging your successes and celebrating your wins can help you realize your worth. You are good enough. You're deserving enough. You're capable enough. You're smart enough, attractive enough, young and old enough. You are strong enough, resourceful enough, resilient, resourceful, and persistent enough. And yes, you're the kind of person who could do something like that. Whatever "that" is for you. You have what it takes to continue to move forward, facing your fears, taking imperfect and uncomfortable action. Sometimes stumbling and falling toward success. Then getting up and trying and perhaps even falling again. Refusing to give up until your reach the goals that are important for you. Yes, there's a lot to celebrate. You are a champion in your own right.

Some people have a hard time celebrating themselves and their own accomplishments. Limiting beliefs about their self-worth and whether they deserve a celebration can get in their way. If you're one of them, it's time to let those go. Even if you started this book with one goal in mind but ended up achieving something else, you deserve credit for reading all the way through to the end. At the very least, you now know that procrastination isn't your fault. You know the reasons you procrastinate and techniques for how to overcome it. You can't unknow what you now know. You now have knowledge and choices. You have planted seeds in your mind that can help you grow into the magnificent achiever you were meant to be. You are now a powerhouse of potential. No one else could have done for you what you just did for yourself.

Please don't wait to celebrate your progress. Celebrate the little successes and milestones all along the way. You don't need to have "arrived" to be happy and enjoy your life. Don't keep putting your happiness off until some point in the future. Don't procrastinate on celebrating you and your efforts and progress to get where you want to go.

Celebrate how far you've come. And celebrate the success you now know how to attain in the future. Let yourself be happy now. Not only does it feel good, but being happy in each moment tends to bring more happiness into your future because as Gandhi and others have noted, what you do today creates your future. If you work on completing your goals each day, you can attain them in your future. Similarly, if you find ways to feel happy today, you are practicing being happy tomorrow. Happiness becomes your comfort zone, something that you automatically create and gravitate toward.

Also, reward yourself. Now is the time to have that special meal at your favorite restaurant. Take a short getaway trip to a fun and relaxing place. Buy yourself a gift, something extra you've been wanting. When I finished writing this book, I bought a new iPhone. I felt like I deserved to pay every penny it cost. Not only did I know I would enjoy using the phone, but I appreciated that it had served as an incentive to dig in and do the work that writing this book required. So splurge on yourself. Light up those dopamine channels. Get in the habit of celebrating after big and small accomplishments. It will make your brain want to achieve even more.

If you didn't make as much progress as you wanted while reading this book, it's never too late for second chances. Re-read the sections you think might be most helpful. Continue to experiment with techniques and strategies you think might work for you. Not only is it not too late, but now you have the knowledge and tools to make up for lost time and move forward even further. Keep going. Keep taking the next step and the next and the next. As long as you don't stop, your success is inevitable. Just knowing that is something to celebrate.

Possible Challenges Ahead

As you continue to overcome your procrastination, circumstances and dynamics in your life will start to change, almost always for the better. But some of those changes may present challenges to navigate. Knowing about them in advance can give you an advantage in how you respond. You'll be better able to anticipate and deal with any challenges you might run into, which will make it easier to keep moving forward.

Please don't get it in your head that these kinds of things WILL happen—only that they MIGHT happen. In other words, don't let these possible challenges become things you expect and therefore, they turn into self-fulfilling prophecies. I'm giving you a heads up about them now in case they show up on your path to success. Knowing about them in advance can keep you from being surprised and thrown off track. As long as you keep moving toward your goals, trust that you can get past the obstacles that get in your way.

If you remember from Chapter Six on goals, Kelly McGonigal found that after teaching classes on willpower to thousands of students at Stanford University, those who had a Plan for Failure were much more likely to succeed. That's because they predicted when, where, and why they might give in and came up with a plan for how they would handle those situations. That's what I'm talking about here. If you can anticipate what future circumstances might cause you to slide back into your procrastination, you will be more likely to successfully overcome them. Not everyone runs into these circumstances. But I'll describe some of the common obstacles you might face.

You can think of these challenges as temporary roadblocks in your movement toward your goals. Just like when you see signs along the road when you're driving that say, "Danger. Hazards ahead." With procrastination, hazards to your forward progress can come from your environment or Outer Game obstacles like time and money. But the hazards I most often see stopping people from success are those from their Inner Game of thoughts, beliefs, and emotions. Here are some of the most common hazards I've seen in myself and others as they journey forward into the life of being a non-procrastinator. Then moving from a non-procrastinator to an achiever.

1. Your Greatest Fear

People often tell me they are afraid to stop procrastinating and finally go after their biggest goals because they're afraid they will fail. That's a valid fear. Failure is always a risk you take when you accept the challenge to go big and play all out. However, many people aren't aware of another fear that often lies underneath their fear of failure, and that's a fear of success. That fear is described by Marianne Williamson in her book *A Return to Love*, where she writes in a piece called "Our Greatest Fear,"

> *Our deepest fear is not that we are inadequate. Our deepest*
> *fear is that we are powerful beyond measure. It is our light*
> *not our darkness that most frightens us.*

In the final analysis, it may not be our fear of failure that scares us the most, but our fear of success and the power of our own potential. But as we continue to overcome our procrastination, and as we face our fears about failure and success, something beautiful begins to happen. Our courage allows us to see our fears for what they are—simply thoughts about things that *might* happen. Maybe those scary things will happen and maybe they won't. Even if they do happen, know that you can find ways around them, just like you have done so often in the past. But you will never know unless you go after what you really want.

Fear can also show up sometimes to keep us safe. Always ask yourself, "What's the worst that could happen?" before trying to move past your fear. Do some problem-solving in advance if you need to. And be aware that holding yourself back because of fears of failure or success may be a possible roadblock along your road toward becoming a non-procrastinator.

2. Your Comfort Zone
Overcoming your procrastination means living more of your life outside your comfort zone. At times, that can feel exhilarating. But when you're finally succeeding and flying high, you're in a new zone that can begin to feel uncomfortable. Some people find it difficult to stay happy and on top of things for very long. If you're one of them, you may look for ways to bring yourself down. You may unconsciously retreat back into your comfort zone of what's normal and familiar. For example, you may start to procrastinate again. Or you may move toward your goals but sabotage your own efforts. In his book *The Big Leap*, author Gay Hendricks describes how you can trigger a form of paralysis whenever you move toward a goal of achieving higher levels of success than you're used to. This paralysis becomes your self-imposed glass ceiling. Your awareness that this *might* happen can help prepare you to handle it if it does.

Another common hazard when you start to live outside your comfort zone is that you will probably bump into the edges of other people's comfort zones, maybe on a regular basis. People may not support you or cheer you on when you succeed or take on big goals—not because you're doing anything wrong but because of their own insecurities. It helps if you can recognize this when it happens. If you need to, go back and read the related section in Chapter Six on how to handle it.

Also, keep in mind there's the possibility that your big goals and efforts to succeed will motivate others instead of trigger their insecurities. There's more to Marianne Williamson's quote from "Our Greatest Fear" which says,

> *And as we let our own light shine, we unconsciously give other*
> *people permission to do the same. As we are liberated from*

our own fear, our presence automatically liberates others.

In other words, the glow from your own light can become a beacon and a source of inspiration for others.

3. Extra Stress

Stress is inevitable. That's because anything that makes demands on us can cause stress, even if those demands come from positive things like getting married or buying a house. Stress is also cumulative. It's that nagging cough that won't go away. It's the conflicts in your relationships. It's not having enough money. Sometimes the demands of life all add up and can overwhelm us. When we go through periods of extra stress, we're more likely to fall back into unhealthy habits and old ways of behavior, which can include procrastination. That means that sometimes,

Under stress, we regress.

When you're under extra stress, your first symptom may be that you're spending more time engaged in your avoidance activities, like more time on your phone. Or you may notice that you're procrastinating because you feel bad emotionally. There's a unique brand of misery that comes from driving with one foot on the gas and one foot on the brakes. You want to move forward, but you're holding back, finding all kinds of reasons and excuses not to do what you want to do and know you should do. The misery that comes from procrastinating is often a combination of guilt, regret, shame, frustration, a sense of helplessness, maybe some confusion, fear, and anger. That misery can be your message, your sign that it's time to start using the techniques you know work to help you get unstuck and move forward. Stay on the lookout for how extra stress can cause you to backslide and can trigger your procrastination. It's a common pitfall.

4. Mistakes and Failures

Even the most successful people make mistakes and flat-out fail. It's not the mistake or slipup that derails you. It's letting that mistake derail you for longer than it needs to for you to learn the lesson your mistake has to teach.

Setbacks from failure or making mistakes often happen when you're already stressed out. You get too tired. You travel and get off your schedule. Unexpected bad news smacks you in the face and sends you into a tailspin. And sometimes, nothing obvious happens to make you fall back into your old ways of procrastinating—you simply give into temptation on one small thing and you start to waiver on your healthy habits.

Maybe you miss one day of exercise, which turns into two and then three days of not working out. Perhaps you've been doing really well with not drinking except on the weekends, but one beer on a Thursday night leads to more steady drinking during the week. Once one domino falls, others are more likely to follow. Have your awareness intact and ready to notice any little slips. Then have a Plan for Failure ready to go so you can recover quickly. Get back on track as fast as you can, before your missteps erode your progress and turn into new habits. A good rule of thumb is that if you slip up and procrastinate once, you'll probably be okay. But if you do the same thing a second time, you can start to build a bad habit, and it may be harder to stop that momentum.

Sometimes people keep failing and making mistakes because they are going after the wrong goal. Or maybe their timing is off and they need to wait for a better time to complete their goal. If you are sure you're on the right path, it might be time to take a break. Pause. But don't stop altogether. Stay curious. Keep exploring. Keep planting bamboo seeds. Wait long enough for the seeds to grow roots under the ground. Stay patient while you continue to prepare yourself for when you do reach your goal and get to enjoy your win.

5. Pre-crastination

Procrastination happens on a continuum. On one end are chronic procrastinators who can't get things done on time (or done at all), and they have lots of problems in their lives. On the other end of the continuum are **pre-crastinators** who can become overly rigid and anxious about getting things done way ahead of time, long before any deadlines. These people can also have problems, although usually less often.

A friend of mine said she always shows up to meetings quite a bit early. When I asked her why she said, "It's part of my perfectionism." Arriving early worked for her. It helped her avoid the stress of being late and of being seen (by herself and others) as imperfect. Plus, other people saw her as dependable and eager to do a good job, which sometimes led to job promotions. Another person told me she was a pre-crastinator, and that it was caused by having to take on a lot of responsibilities in her family when she was a young girl. Her way of coping was to become a perfectionist and a pre-crastinator, which worked while she was in her family but it caused problems in her adult life. She made decisions so early that she often changed her mind several times before it was time to decide. That sometimes caused stress for her and others when everyone had to keep changing their plans.

Be careful about becoming a pre-crastinator. The goal is to get to a point in your life where you have a CHOICE. You can choose to wait to complete a task, especially when that is a strategic technique, used at times when waiting is the best thing to do. You can also get something done well ahead of time, mark it off your to-do list, and move ahead in your life, feeling good about already having it completed. I hope you can get to a point of giving yourself a choice.

6. Misinterpreting Your Struggles

Many of our big goals, the ones that challenge us the most, have hard parts. For starters, aspects of achieving those goals often require lots of hard work. At times, we may feel frustrated or unsure about what to do next. We may make mistakes and have to try many different approaches before we finally get it right and reach our goals. All of this is perfectly normal. Our most important goals often require struggle. Lots of struggle.

However, many people misinterpret the struggle. They may ask themselves, "How can something that seems like such an important goal be so hard to accomplish? Am I doing this all wrong? Is something wrong with me? Why can't I figure this out?" But here's the deal. The struggle may be necessary. It's often part of the process of finally breaking free from the constraints of your old ways of doing things. The struggle forces you to stretch and grow, to learn new habits and skills that will be necessary when you improve your life and move to higher ground, when you move out of your comfort zone and into new, unexplored territory. It's all part of the learning process. As long as you don't quit, your struggles can eventually give you strength.

Here's an analogy. Caterpillars must go through tremendous struggle in order to break free from their cocoons and become butterflies. Struggling to get out of the cocoon is what builds enough strength in their wings for them to fly when they finally emerge. Without this self-sustaining strength in their wings, the caterpillars will quickly perish. Plus, each caterpillar needs to go through this struggle by itself. No one else can help it avoid the struggle or make it easier. In other words, there is a purpose and a reason for the struggle. It makes the wings form correctly and allows the caterpillar to turn into a butterfly and begin a new journey in the world.

The same is often true for each of us. It may be difficult to go through your own struggles. You may get discouraged and want to quit. But your struggles may be what allow you to eventually move out of your old ways of doing things and into new territory, places where you can soar to new heights of achievement and enjoyment. Your struggles can be a rite of passage to the land of freedom—but only *after* you have developed enough strength to break free from your comfort zone. This process reminds me of a motivational poster at my gym that says,

Sore today, soar tomorrow.

Sometimes the struggles we go through are exactly what we need.

Be on the lookout though for times when your struggle is self-created and you're making things harder than they need to be. For example, sometimes we try to change and control things in our lives that we have no control over. In these situations, it's often best to start with acceptance. Then look for ways to take response-ability for changing your reaction to the situation. Or sometimes we struggle unnecessarily because we believe it *should* be hard. Or maybe we're worrying about all the details of how we will achieve a goal, when all we need to do is keep moving forward and the details will fall into place. The point is to be careful about how you interpret your struggles.

7. Those sticky, tricky, and sometimes ridiculously stubborn limiting beliefs

The most common hazard I see when people can't seem to make progress on their goals, despite what looks like sincere effort, is limiting beliefs. It's the obstacle I look for first, because around eight times out of ten, it's this internal block that's holding people back. Many people keep trying different Outer Game techniques to reach their goals, but without success. In other words, they **try to solve an internal problem by using external solutions**. Or if they do have some success, it takes forever and requires a tremendous amount of effort. Or sometimes they succeed, but quickly lose what they gained, like when people win the lottery but end up bankrupt in a few years. This quote from Robert W. Service expresses it well,

It isn't the mountain ahead that wears you out; it's the grain of sand in your shoe.

Sometimes this failure pattern is due to not enough effort. Not enough persistence. Not enough resourcefulness to figure out the right combination of techniques for success. And on rare occasions, it's due to bad timing. The timing isn't right to achieve a particular goal. Once you're aware of this possibility, you can often realize that it might be better to wait and do something later rather than sooner. Or possibly not do it at all. Remember, sometimes what looks like procrastination is our intuition telling us *not* to do something. However, this can be risky, because you don't want to use these unusual possibilities as justification to procrastinate.

Sometimes you may try to reach your goals, but when you don't achieve them by the time you think you should, you fall into a hidden limiting belief that you'll never succeed. That you'll never have whatever it takes to be successful, including the time and energy. Remember, you can always get back on track, continue to move toward your goal, and find that you have plenty of time and energy to succeed. In fact, usually more than enough.

I'm not saying it won't be hard to get around the dangerous hazards you encounter, perhaps especially your limiting beliefs. At times, your journey may be extremely hard. Here's a powerful affirmation to use when you get stuck. I heard this from Lauren O'Connell on her YouTube video on "Aging Well" and it really rang true for me.

I can do hard things.
This is a hard thing and I can do it.

This can be your mantra, your power phrase when things get especially tough. It's not an over-the-top positive affirmation about your strength and might. Just a simple acknowledgement that things are hard—and you can do hard things. When you repeatedly tell yourself you can do hard things—and you watch yourself doing them—it starts to override any beliefs that you're not up to the challenge or you're not good enough, in whatever ways you believe that to be true. (This is a slightly different version of author Glennon Doyle's quote that says, "These things will be hard to do, but you can do hard things." In this case, using the word "I" seems to make it more powerful.)

That's not to say your pesky limiting beliefs won't continue to pop up and have the potential to stop you in your tracks, both when you're aware of them and when you're not. They often stick around and get in the way of our progress even when we know what they are. For example, even knowing my two main limiting beliefs are *Don't be too powerful* and *Don't outshine others*, they sometimes still drift through my mind when I try to reach my big goals. Knowing what they are helps me get around them. So does remembering this story.

According to Cherokee legend, an elder grandfather told his grandson there is a battle going on inside all people. He said, "This battle is between two wolves. One wolf is Fear. The wolf of Fear carries anxiety, uncertainty, doubt, indecision, and inaction. The other wolf is Faith. The wolf of Faith brings calm, commitment, enthusiasm, confidence, decisiveness, and action. This same battle is going on inside of you."

The grandson took a moment to reflect on this and then asked, "Which wolf will win?"

The grandfather simply replied, "The one you feed."

The moral of this story is to be aware of your thoughts—those that create fear and those that instill trust and faith. Ignore your limiting thoughts and beliefs. Let them drift by like clouds in the sky. Or challenge the thoughts. They may not even be true. You can also counter your limiting thoughts with positive affirmations. Focus your attention on empowering thoughts that give you the faith and courage to move forward in your life.

I ran into every one of these seven hazards on my way toward writing and publishing this book. Every single one. Sometimes it was rough. But I kept plugging along, knowing deep in my heart that publishing this book was too big of a dream to abandon. Despite lots of setbacks and mistakes—and tons of frustration—I kept taking the next step and the next and the next.

Then something unexpected happened. I started to fear NOT achieving my goal more than I feared achieving it. I started to fear getting to the end of my life and feeling deep regret that I didn't push through the challenges and publish this book. That fear became a gift of motivation. I was so scared I *wouldn't* achieve my goal that I was willing to go through the frustrations and failures of what I now know are a normal part of stretching yourself to achieve something that's way outside your comfort zone. Something that brings you face to face with whatever is inside of you that would cause you to quit. Facing your fears and inner demons is incredibly empowering. Probably one of the most empowering things you can do.

Now when I think about achieving some of my other big goals, there's a little fear, knowing it will be scary to move out of my comfort zone and into the unknown. But the bigger fear I have is thinking that I *won't* achieve my goals, that I'll find excuses or get sidetracked in other directions. That I'll regret copping out, and that I'll have to live with that regret for the rest of my life. No thanks.

Many of us will continue to face limiting beliefs about how high we can fly and how far we can go with our success. If that happens to you, don't let those beliefs stop you from moving forward. If you keep using the techniques that work for you, if you give yourself lots of rewards and self-care along the way, and if you make sure to get enough support from others, there are no limits to your potential and the opportunities that are waiting for you to enjoy.

Imagine This! You As Your Best Self

Now that you are aware of the hazards that might trip you up as you continue to overcome your procrastination, you are much better prepared to prevent that from happening. You are aware of potential obstacles in the road ahead, and that awareness becomes your strength and your protection going forward.

At the beginning of this book, I suggested that you get a picture of one goal you wanted to achieve by the time you finished your reading. I mentioned that if you completed that goal, it would indicate you understood why you procrastinate, you had mastered new skills to stop procrastinating, and you'd become more productive in general, at least enough to get you moving toward your goals instead of away from them. Not only that, but the skills you would develop along the way were skills you could use for the rest of your life. All those outcomes are more reasons to celebrate.

Now that you have finished the book, I would like to leave you with another picture in your head. This will be a picture of you going forward in your life as a non-procrastinator. As someone who has successfully navigated the internal and external obstacles that have held you back in the past from being your best self. None of us has arrived yet, and none of us need to try to be perfect. We are all works in progress throughout our lives. This new picture, though, will be a snapshot of your Future Self as you continue to overcome your procrastination and enjoy the positive results of your achievements. It will be a mental picture of what you ideally want your life to look like.

Take about 15 minutes to be alone and have a pen and paper available so you can do some writing afterward. You can read through this imagery activity and let your imagination go free while you read. You can also record this activity on your phone and listen to your recording with your eyes closed. Listening to your own voice as it guides you through this exercise can be especially powerful. Whether you're reading this activity or listening to a recording, start by sitting quietly in a comfortable position. Take a few slow, deep breaths. On each exhale, imagine that you are letting go of any stress, worry, or tension. Keep breathing like this until you feel completely relaxed.

Now imagine that you can jump forward into the future and see (in your mind) what your life might look like during an ideal day, when you've developed healthy habits to overcome your procrastination and have already completed many of your longer-term goals. You will go through this ideal day as your best self. As the best version of yourself. As the non-procrastinator who already lives inside of you. As you read or listen to these descriptions and questions, *see* the pictures of your answers in your mind and *feel* your answers as if they have already become your new reality. Also *hear* any sounds in your environment or maybe a voice in your head that is positive and supports you as you go through your ideal day. Take your time. There's no rush. Allow yourself plenty of time to answer each of the questions silently, in your mind.

To get started, imagine you are first waking up in the morning on your ideal day. You immediately notice you feel rested, energized, and excited about what will happen during this day. As you look around your bedroom, you become aware that you love the colors in the room and the way the room is designed and decorated. You become aware you feel the same way about the rest of your house, because of how it looks and how it makes you feel to live here. Where is your ideal house located? Do you live in a city? In the country? Near a beach? In the mountains? What would be the best house and the best location for your house in your ideal future?

As you begin your day, notice what you do first. Do you have a morning routine that starts your day, with a focus on activities that help you stay physically and mentally fit? What are those activities? Do you exercise, meditate, write in a journal, or count your blessings? Imagine you have chosen activities that help set the tone for your day to be ideal in every way.

Next, imagine that you are starting into your morning and what you will do during your morning hours. How will you spend your time? Will you work? Will you play? Will you do both? Do you have a job? If so, do you work in your house or outside your house? If you have a job, become aware of how enjoyable and fulfilling it is to work at that job. You're grateful it also provides plenty of financial rewards, making sure you have all the financial freedom you want.

As you go about your day, you notice things happen that used to distract you from what you planned to do, distractions that used to lead to procrastination. But now, you catch those distractions right away and prevent them from interfering with your plans. Your awareness is razor sharp, and it continues to support your healthy lifestyle, one where you can stick to your schedule and do what's important and enjoyable for you. You no longer use your energy against yourself. You no longer sabotage your own plans and goals. Instead, you use your time and energy to create the life you want. And for that, you are immensely thankful.

Also notice how you spend your free time. Do you enjoy spending time with your family, being active in sports, or focused on hobbies like traveling, cooking, or reading? Who are your friends and what kinds of activities do you enjoy doing together? What are you passionate about? Become aware of how grateful you are to yourself for finding your passion and purpose and making those a priority. You know that spending time doing the things you're passionate about makes you feel alive and makes your life feel richer and more fulfilling. You've also learned that taking the time to focus on your health and living a healthy lifestyle means you get to feel good physically in your ideal future.

Now imagine it's the end of your ideal day, and you are getting ready to go to sleep. Do you have an evening routine that helps you wrap up that day and prepare for the next one? If so, what activities do you include in your evening routine? Maybe you identify at least one win, something you did well during your day and can feel proud about. Maybe you identify at least one thing you're grateful for in your life. For example, you may feel grateful that procrastination is no longer a problem for you, which opens the door for so many other blessings to fill your life. Blessings like more time and energy to do the things you want, better health, greater financial wealth, and new-found levels of happiness. The gratitude and positive feelings you feel right before you go to sleep stay with you all through the night, helping you sleep better and wake up refreshed, feeling positive and eager to head into another ideal day, one that could be even better.

Once you've had a chance to see, feel, and hear your ideal day sometime in the future, then once again focus on your breathing. Notice how you are sitting. When you're ready, open your eyes if they have been closed and return to the present. Next, find the pen and paper you placed nearby before you began. Take as long as you need to write down what you learned from doing that imagery activity. Write down what you want to remember from your experience. Information that comes from your imagination can quickly fade from memory, so it's important to write it down immediately. You also might want to thank yourself for taking the time to do this imagery. The pictures in your head about your future become a guiding light in where and how your life unfolds. Perhaps sooner than you think, your current life may begin to match the ideal day you just imagined.

You Were Born to Shine

Have you ever asked yourself some of the big questions in life? Questions like, "Who am I?" and "Why am I here?" "What's my purpose?" And "Am I on the right path?" As we get further into adulthood, most of us eventually start to wonder about these questions. Searching for the answers can lead to discovering deeper parts of yourself.

I believe we are here for a reason. We have lessons to learn, dreams to achieve, a purpose to fulfill, and this phenomenal lifelong opportunity to develop our potential and share our gifts and talents with the world. As we learn our lessons, and as we begin to accomplish our mission and fulfill our purpose, we automatically start to become the brightest and best version of ourselves. Our authentic ideal selves. The self who is continually developing more and more of our potential. The self who not only shines in their own life, but is whose light is so bright that it shines on others and enriches their lives as well.

I agree with author Eckard Tolle who says we all have two purposes in life, an **inner purpose** and an **outer purpose**.

1. **Our inner purpose is about BEING**. It's about continually learning and growing mentally, emotionally, and spiritually, which allows you to reach more and more of your unlimited potential. Your mission this lifetime, should you choose to accept it, is to *be* the best, the healthiest, the most loving, and the most authentic version of yourself. All of us share this same purpose.

2. **Our outer purpose is about DOING**. Each of us came into this world with talents and gifts that are unique to us. Just as no two grains of sand

are exactly alike, each of us is one of a kind. Our outer purpose is to discover and develop our one-of-a-kind talents and gifts and share them with the world. In *doing* that, we naturally fulfill more and more of our inner purpose to be our best selves.

If you're not living the purposeful life you're meant to live, and if you're not happy with your life as it is right now, then ask yourself, "What's stopping me? What's keeping me from going after what would make me truly happy?" People often respond to those questions with things like, "If I change my life, it might not work out." Or "I could end up worse than where I started." These are normal fears. But you don't need to let those fears stop you from exploring different and better ways to live. It may be time to at least begin to think of your ideal future, a future where you would feel authentic, purposeful, plugged in, and alive. A future where you had a meaningful reason to get up every morning, looking forward to what you had planned for the day. Just like you did when you imagined your ideal future during the imagery activity earlier in this chapter.

I see so many people in the world who seem lost, with no real purpose for why they are here. Without that purpose and guiding light in their lives, they wander around going from one dopamine high to another, getting as much pleasure out of every moment as they can, but without an end-goal in mind. They don't see the big picture for their lives. They want to enjoy life and be happy, but they find that enjoyment and happiness through high-dopamine activities that don't add much value to their lives. And sadly, it's mostly because they don't know they have choices.

Too much dopamine for too much of the time cuts them off from themselves. They can't stay connected to themselves, their own values, and the kind of person they want to be, much less discover the mission they want to accomplish during their lives. I feel like we're living in "The Land of the Lost" where, as Henry David Thoreau said, far too many people "lead lives of quiet desperation."

It doesn't have to be that way for you. You now know how to tap into your body's own natural neurochemicals to feel good most of the time—while doing valuable activities—and without the cost of overloading your brain with too much dopamine. By using the flow state and by learning how to use techniques like the Inner Witness, you can learn how to ride a natural high through most of your life, just like Brian Tracy has done. If you remember, Tracy has led a highly productive life, writing more than 70 books and speaking to over five million people around the world. He attributes his productivity and natural high to brain chemicals that get triggered when you get into the habit of starting and finishing important jobs. While you're feeling this natural high, the valuable activities you're doing can not only enrich your life, but also the lives of others. It all starts with knowing you have choices.

Is it possible for the rest of us to develop this "positive addiction" the same way Tracy has? The neuroscientist Candace Pert says, "Yes." As we discussed, she's the person who discovered that emotions are chemical molecules in our brains and bodies and concluded that because of these molecules, we're hardwired to live in natural states of bliss. People often look for shortcuts to these blissful states by taking mind-altering drugs and doing other things that blast their brains with too much dopamine. Those shortcuts always have downsides and are never as high or as pure as tapping into your body's natural ability to create these blissful states.

Developing a habit of starting and finishing important jobs will give you better chances to feel naturally high most of the time. So will knowing your purpose in life. Besides becoming your best self, do you know your life purpose? At least one thing you're meant to do during your life? If you haven't yet discovered your external purpose and reason for being here, it's never too late. Ask yourself these questions.

- What are my strengths, my unique talents and gifts?
- What am I naturally good at?
- What makes me feel good about myself and proud of myself?
- What makes me feel more connected in healthy ways to other people?
- What is a healthy activity I would love doing all day long, even if I didn't get paid for it?
- What do I really enjoy and am good at that could benefit other people as well?
- What is my passion? What feeds my soul?

You can start with those questions. If your answers to those questions don't quite ring true, then ask,

- What am I interested in? What am I curious about?
- How do I spend my free time?
- What did I enjoy doing as a kid?

If you still feel stumped, go back to the writing you did in Chapter Six on goals, where you answered this question about your top five wishes.

- What five things would I need to accomplish in order to feel successful at the end of my life? Then ask yourself what one of two of those five things you could start to focus on now.

Your answers to these questions can start to point you in the direction of your talents and gifts. If you're still not sure, then guess. What's your best guess about your greatest strength, what you're naturally good at? Often it's something that's hiding in plain sight. Keep questioning. Keep exploring. Try out different possibilities. Volunteer and get some experience at what you think *might* be your purpose. Also, know that your purpose can be expressed in different ways. For example, I love helping people change for the better. It's one of the most rewarding things I can do. Throughout my life, I've helped people change in different ways— through teaching, counseling, coaching, and now, through my writing.

Like many others, I have found that decisions are easier to make when they are guided by asking, "Will this support my purpose?" Besides that, knowing my purpose gives me more focus, energy, and drive, especially when it is bigger than me and involves helping others. When you find your purpose—your reason to get going every day—you find meaning in your own life and at the same time, help to make the world a better place. Sharing your gifts and talents is one of the best life purposes you can find. There's nothing quite like the reward and fulfillment that comes from using your gifts in ways that make a difference in the lives of others.

Knowing my purpose has also accelerated my progress toward building the life I want. Lots of studies have been done with people who have found meaning and purpose in their lives. Those studies consistently show that having a life purpose improves your mental and physical health, enhances resiliency, enhances self-esteem, decreases the chances of depression, increases overall well-being and life satisfaction, and increases life expectancy for both younger and older adults. In other words, having a purpose works wonders for your health. These benefits also help provide the abundant energy and positive mindset that can help you to reach your loftiest goals.

One of the most astounding and exciting parts of this whole puzzle in life is this: once you find your unique gift and offer it to others as only you can—if others want your gift or have a need for your gift—it can become your job, your career, your source of income. There's always the possibility you can find ways to get paid for doing what you love. That you can make a difference in other people's lives as you're doing it. Sharing your gift with the world becomes a life purpose that brings blessings to you and others at the same time. One of the essential keys to getting started is to move beyond procrastination. Once you overcome that obstacle, the rest of the puzzle pieces will start to fall into place.

Find a Way

You may remember from the news that in 2013, Diana Nyad became the first person to swim from Cuba to Florida—without a shark cage. This 110-mile channel is one of the most treacherous water passages in the world. Nyad had tried four times before to swim the distance, but the dangers had always prevented her success. She finally did it when she was sixty-four years old. In doing that, Nyad fulfilled her own life dream and became an inspiration, role model, and source of motivation for millions of others.

After so many unsuccessful attempts, Nyad knew the dangers all too well. On her fifth attempt, she planned for each and every one of them. These dangers included not only sharks, but the cold temperatures of the water. Currents, which could shift and make her swim longer and harder. The scorching sun. The sheer physical stamina needed to go the distance, without sleep. The mental fortitude required to pull off such a monumental feat.

Nyad's previous experiences told her she could probably overcome those obstacles with proper training and support from her team of assistants. But the biggest obstacle she faced was from the poisonous box jellyfish that had stopped one of her previous attempts. The toxins from their stings are the most deadly and fast-acting in the entire animal kingdom. People who get stung while they are in the ocean often die before they make it to shore. Nyad knew if she didn't anticipate that obstacle, her dream would never come true.

So she dug in. She made a commitment not only to anticipate the jellyfish, but to do everything she could to prevent their stings from robbing her of success. She hired a company to make a special body suit that would allow for free movement but also protect her skin from stings. She hired another company to make a protective face mask. She practiced swimming in both. She asked for adjustments to the fabrics and fit. She practiced some more. Finally, she found what she hoped would protect her.

Preparing for jellyfish was part of Nyad's Plan for Failure, and it worked. She successfully completed her swim in 53 hours, without stopping. Her swim received news coverage around the world. Millions of people were inspired by her motivation, her perseverance, her inner strength, and her determination to reach her goal in spite of the difficulties and obstacles that could have held her back.

Nyad's training also included a focus on the mental fortitude she knew she would need. She used a mantra to get her through the hardest of the hard parts: *Find a way*. That mantra was her cue to dig deeper inside of herself when the going got tough. To become more resourceful than she ever had been in the past. To use all her strengths to somehow find the resiliency to recover from all her past failures. To be persistent and keep going no matter what. To know and believe that she was enough. That she had done enough. She was strong enough and smart enough to succeed. That knowing and those beliefs provided a foundation for her belief that she *could* find a way. That she could succeed. That her dream could become a reality. It was a dream that had lived in her heart for 35 years.

After her swim, Nyad wrote a book called *Find a Way*, which can provide motivation for even the least motivated among us. In case you're interested, there's also a movie being made about her called "Nyad" that promises to be beyond inspiring. In many ways we are all like Diana. Swimming through our lives, facing obstacles and difficulties along the way. Hopefully, learning from our failures so we can eventually reach the distant shore of our own dreams. Giving our all to how we live our lives each day.

One of the most important lessons Diana learned from her successful swim is that **completing an especially difficult goal changes you. It changes who you are as a person**. Diana was a different person after her successful swim. Stronger. More confident. More satisfied with herself. More at peace. When we complete a goal that was particularly challenging, we develop more of our potential. We step it up a notch and become more of the person we were born to be. We change into more of the best version of ourselves. Achieving whatever goal helped us do that is just a bonus. The real value is the personal growth because that opens the door and helps us prepare for even greater accomplishments in the future. We move into a place where "more" is possible. More choices, motivation, and inspiration. You start to develop a **more mindset**, realizing you are meant for more.

I'm not referring to more material possessions that can clutter your life and weigh you down, although those are fine if you enjoy them. I'm referring to the things we can welcome into our lives that will make them richer, more meaningful, and more enjoyable on a deeper level. Like more love. More abundance. More income, freedom, and health. A deeper sense of purpose and fulfillment. You open yourself up to the endless possibilities that come when you say to yourself, "I'm here to be more, do more, and give more."

We all go through the same process as Diana did when we start to overcome our procrastination. Here's how Henry David Thoreau expressed it,

What you get by achieving your goals is not as important as what you become by achieving your goals.

You become a different person when you make a firm commitment to stop procrastinating. It sets off a cascade of changes in who you are as a person. Your core identity changes. Your core identity is what determines much of your behavior. This process happens naturally as you continue to do what it takes, to take imperfect and uncomfortable action toward reaching your goals and fulfilling your dreams.

What drove Diana to push herself that long and hard? What was her motivation? As she describes in her book, she always wanted to be the kind of person who never, ever gives up. Someone who pushes herself to give every ounce of what she's got to her dream and to the way she lives her life. And who in the end, has no regrets. It's an intrinsic motivation that has influenced every day of her adult life and caused her to far surpass the standards others usually set for themselves.

However, Diana also realized that as Winston Churchill said, "Never give in except to convictions of honour and good sense." In other words, don't keep going toward a goal if it compromises your integrity or if due to circumstances, it no longer makes sense. Diana abandoned her goal four times when circumstances like jellyfish stings forced her to stop. But her dream lived on inside of her, and she kept trying until she finally made it.

What Kind of Person Do You Want to Be?

I don't know about you, but when I stop to think about it, I want to be the kind of person I admire and respect. Someone who says what they mean and means what they say. Someone who walks my talk. Someone who has integrity, who honors their promises to themselves and others. If I say I'm going to do something, I do it, unless circumstances tell me not to. I want to be the kind of person who is courageous enough to take on my big goals and persistent enough to do what it takes to achieve them. Someone who is a hard worker, who digs in when the going gets tough. Someone who becomes even more resourceful when faced with obstacles and never gives up on my dreams. Someone who believes in myself and my infinite capacity for love and joy. Someone who is kind and generous with myself in the ways I talk to myself and care for myself. Someone who is also kind and generous with other people and looks for ways to help others and lift them up. I have a long way to go to reach that ideal image of myself. But at least I have a picture of the ideal person I want to be.

What about you? What kind of person do you want to be? What values do you hold? Who would you want to be in order to feel happy and proud of yourself? I encourage you to jot down at least five values or characteristics that describe your ideal Future Self and who you want to become.

But here's the deal. We can't become our best selves if we continue to procrastinate. Whenever you're tempted to check your phone instead of focusing on your goals, remember what kind of person you want to be. Each time you're about to reach for that junk food, think about the habits of the healthy person you aspire to become. If you want to quit and give up on your goals when they get hard, remind yourself that you're now the kind of person who keeps going when the going gets tough. Remember your values and the picture you have of your best self. You can use that image to help you avoid procrastination and stay on track with your plans.

It's usually easy to tap into the extrinsic motivation of wanting to reach your goals. You're motivated to do things like get fit, take that dream vacation, and make more money. But by seeing yourself as the best version of yourself, you can also tap into the intrinsic motivation of feeling good about who you are as a person. Both of these sources of motivation can combine to give you extra strength and courage to achieve goals you never thought were possible. They connect you to the most basic of all human motivations to seek pleasure, which is a DNA-driven resource we can use in healthy ways. With awareness, we can also prevent ourselves from using our desire for pleasure in unhealthy ways.

There is no failure if you have given your best effort. You can always hold your head up high and feel proud of yourself if you live each day, doing the best you can. A part of you already knows that if you do that, when you get to the end of your life, you will have no regrets. You can look back on the time you had here and feel happy and proud that you took advantage of the opportunities your life had to offer.

When people who are at the end of their lives are asked about their biggest regrets, here's what they say: it's not what they did—but what they *didn't* do—that they regret the most. When you overcome your procrastination, you can keep yourself from being among those people. You can save yourself from living a life of regrets. Like Diana Nyad, find a way. Just keep going until your reach your goals, until you achieve the success you've dreamed about. Become the non-procrastinator who already lives inside of you.

You now know that procrastination isn't your fault and never was. The fault was in your approach, in the *way* or *ways* you had tried to stop procrastinating before. You needed different strategies in order to get the results you wanted. This book contains strategies that can help you finally stop procrastinating and start living your life as an achiever. Happier. Healthier. Wealthier.

You're the only one who can figure out which strategies will work for you. No one else can do that for you, just like no one else can do your push-ups for you. But you have the persistence, resourcefulness, and resilience to do that for yourself. Your hidden power to succeed is no longer hidden. You now have the knowledge and skills to finally stop procrastinating and make your dreams come true.

Tell yourself you will find a way. Listen to your inner voice, the one that's positive, hopeful, encouraging, and supportive. Keep going until you reach your dreams. And know that I'll be cheering you on, every step of the way.

Your future is incredibly bright. It's time to step into your light.

Find a way.

Chapter 10 Highlights

You made it! You're at the end of the last chapter of this book. Consider yourself a warrior. A hero. A champion in your own right. Only a small percentage of people read books at all, and very few of them read an entire book. Your stick-to-itiveness is definitely a cause for celebration.

Now you have the information you need to become the shining light you are meant to be. You've got this. Don't give up. No more procrastinating.

No more holding back. In order to do that, here are more main points to keep in mind.

1. We all have two purposes in life, an **inner purpose** and an **outer purpose**. Our inner purpose is about BEING the best and most authentic version of ourselves. Our outer purpose is about DOING. It's about discovering and developing our talents and gifts and sharing those with others.

2. When you find your unique gifts and offer those to others—if they have a need or a desire for your gifts—your gifts and strengths can become your job, your career, your source of income. There's always the possibility you can find ways to get paid for doing what you love. That you can make a difference in other people's lives as you're doing it.

3. When you get into the habit of starting and finishing important jobs, it triggers brain chemicals that create a natural high. By focusing on important jobs, and by using techniques like flow and the Inner Witness, you can learn how to spend most of your time in a state of happiness and bliss.

4. Discovering your purpose in life can provide motivation and inspiration to live a life without regrets. One of the essential keys to getting started is to move from procrastination to achievement. Once you learn that process, the rest of the puzzle pieces will start to fall into place.

Action Steps

1. Celebrate reading to the end of this book. Light up your dopamine channels by giving yourself a reward or two. Celebrations and rewards will make your brain want to achieve even more.

2. Be cautious of common challenges as you become a non-procrastinator, an achiever. These challenges or hazards include fear of success, misinterpreting your struggles, and backsliding when you make mistakes or you're under extra stress.

3. Do the imagery activity and imagine an ideal day in your future, a day when you have overcome your procrastination and are living life as your best self. The pictures in your head about your ideal future become a guiding light for where and how your life unfolds.

4. If you intended to make more progress while reading this book than you actually did, it's never too late to succeed. Re-read the sections you think might be the most helpful. Continue to experiment with strategies you think might work for you. As long as you continue to move forward, to

find a way, your success is inevitable.

5. Become your own cheerleader, your own coach, using your positive thoughts and self-talk to cheer yourself on as you continue your journey toward overcoming your procrastination and becoming a stunningly successful achiever. Just as I have done throughout this book, give yourself generous amounts of praise and encouragement by telling yourself things like, "Good job. Way to go! Hang in there. You've got this. You're so close. Just keep going. You can make it."

Next Steps

Now that you have finished reading this book, where do you go from here? What are some next steps you might consider? If you start to struggle with your procrastination, I encourage you to continue to experiment with the techniques in this book and keep practicing the ones that work for you. You might also want to read other books on related topics. A recommended reading list is included in the next few pages.

I also suggest that you visit my website at lindagannaway.com where you will find this free resource:

20 Powerful Affirmations for Health, Wealth, and Happiness

This list not only gives you 20 powerful and compelling affirmations. It also includes suggestions for how to use these affirmations to change your thinking and your life in phenomenal ways.

FINALLY Stop Procrastinating Online Course

Coming soon! I am also planning to offer an online course based on this book. The course will help you learn how to apply the techniques, tips, and tools in your own life and get even better at overcoming your procrastination. But this course is unlike most other online courses. Instead, it turns learning into a game, where you earn points and get rewarded—with dopamine! When you slack off, it gently reminds you that you haven't been active in a while and encourages you to get back in the game. People who take these kinds of online courses report that they are fun, engaging and yes, almost "addictive." But this can be a healthy addiction because when you stop procrastinating, you can improve your life across the board. Stay tuned! If you visit my website and request any of the free resources, I will have your email address and will contact you when the online course is available.

You're Invited

Please let me hear from you! I love hearing how people are doing with the material in this book—both your successes and wins and your not-yet successes. All of it is part of the learning process. You may reach me through my website at lindagannaway.com.

Sharing the information in this book is my passion and my calling. Please keep me in mind if you need a speaker or trainer for your group or organization.

I'm on a mission to help as many people as I can with the information in this book. You're invited to be a part of that. If you found this book helpful, please spread the word that there are techniques that even the most die-hard procrastinators can use to finally start getting things done. Here are some ways to share the good news:

- Write a review on Amazon.

- Tell any procrastinators you know about this book. Or better yet, give them a copy (they might procrastinate on buying a copy for themselves!).

- If the book has helped you, share that on social media.

- Look for opportunities to help people who keep putting things off, especially important things, like taking care of their health.

- If you are a member of a book club, suggest this book as one of your selections. The Discussion Guide in the next few pages lists some questions that can help your members understand and overcome their needless delays. Talking about your procrastination with others is a great way to increase your own ability to succeed.

No one is immune from the tricky time thief that can rob us of our health, our wealth, and our happiness. But with awareness and the right strategies, we can each create the successful future we deserve.

Recommended Reading

Here are some suggestions for further reading. Remember, the more you know about the areas in your life where you're stuck, the better your chances for improvement. Your knowledge and understanding can help you get unstuck and achieve your goals faster and easier. So I encourage you to keep reading. This list of books will give you a good place to start.

To get more information on each book, find the book on Amazon and read the description. You can also click on the "Read Sample" feature and read through the table of contents and sample material. That should give you a pretty good idea of whether it's a book you might want to read.

PROCRASTINATION

1. *Eat That Frog* by Brian Tracy

2. *How to Beat Procrastination in the Digital Age* by Linda Sapadin

3. *The Procrastination Equation* by Piers Steel

4. *Stop Procrastinating* by Nils Salzgeber

SPECIFIC TECHNIQUES FOR OVERCOMING PROCRASTINATION

1. *Abundance Unleashed* by Christian Mickelsen

2. *Goodbye, Hurt and Pain* by Deborah Sandella

3. *Letting Go* by David Hawkins

GOAL SETTING

1. *The Willpower Instinct* by Kelly McGonigal

2. *Principles for Success (10th Anniversary Edition)* by Jack Canfield

3. *Goals!* by Brian Tracy

CHANGING YOUR HABITS

1. *The Power of Habits* by Charles Duhigg

2. *Atomic Habits* by James Clear

3. *Tiny Habits* by B.J. Fogg

OVERCOMING INTERNET ADDICTION

1. *Dopamine Nation* by Anna Lembke

2. *How to Break Up with Your Phone* by Rebecca Price

3. *Irresistible* by Adam Alter

TIME MANAGEMENT

1. *The Rise of Superman* by Steven Kotler (includes information on flow)

2. *The One Thing* by Gary Keller and Jay Papasan

3. *Millionaire Success Habits* by Dean Graziosi

MOTIVATION

1. *Find a Way* by Diana Nyad

2. *Believe It!* by Jamie Kern Lima

FINALLY Stop Procrastinating Discussion Guide

Now that you've finished reading this book, I hope you will continue to think about the ideas, experiment with the techniques, and identify the lessons you learn. You can also share your lessons, comments, and questions with family members, friends, and coworkers. If you're a member of a book club, the following 20 questions can help guide your group discussion. You can also ask and answer these questions just with yourself. They will help you stay involved with the material and gain even more from your reading.

1. What is the most important takeaway you learned from this book? What makes that important to you?

2. Think back to the first time you remember procrastinating or one of the first times. What was the situation? What happened after you procrastinated? If other people were involved, how did they react? How did you feel after you procrastinated?

3. Think about what you learned from your first procrastination experience. Maybe you learned that you would get in trouble for your delays. Or maybe you learned that you could get away with it, even though there might be an emotional price to pay. What lesson(s) did you learn from the first time you remember putting something off?

4. Before reading this book, did you think of yourself as a **situational procrastinator** because you procrastinated in only a few areas of your life? Or did you see yourself as more of a **chronic procrastinator** because you procrastinated in many areas of your life and couldn't manage to stop? Share details for your answer.

5. What have been the consequences of your procrastination? Frustration? Guilt? Regret? Overwhelm? Feeling like a failure? Those are internal consequences. What about external consequences like missed opportunities or people getting mad at you? Identify at least three internal consequences and three external consequences that have resulted from your delays.

6. Do you know other procrastinators—maybe friends, coworkers, or family members? How do you feel toward them, especially if their procrastination affects you? Do you feel less judgmental toward other

procrastinators after reading this book? Whether you do or don't feel less judgmental, explain why.

7. Identify and share any areas of your life or any activities where you are still procrastinating. What do you think will be your biggest regret(s) in the future if you continue to put these off?

8. Before you read this book, did you spend too much time on your cell phone or on the internet? Has the amount of time you spend online changed because of reading this book? If so, how? Identify any current concerns you have about your screen time.

9. Do you have concerns about the amount of time any of your friends or family members spend on their screens? If so, have you talked with them about that? Would you consider talking with them about that? Why or why not?

10. When you were reading this book, did you figure out what reward or payoff you were getting from your procrastination? Maybe a feeling of power within yourself or power over other people? Maybe simply a way to avoid feeling uncomfortable? Once you know the reward for your procrastination, you can look for healthy ways to get that need or desire met. What are two healthy ways you can get your needs met instead of procrastinating?

11. All procrastinators have a "procrastination story." It includes the history of their procrastination and the internal and external consequences. But your story isn't over yet. You can always make up a "happy ending"—a positive way for your procrastination story to end. If you haven't already, make up a happy ending, then share your procrastination story and your happy ending with at least one other person. Also, say your happy ending often to yourself.

12. At the end of Chapter Two you learned how to use sports psychology to help you achieve your goals. This technique includes seeing, hearing, and feeling your success before you actually accomplish your goals. If you did that activity, what was it like? Do you think it made your goals easier to achieve? Consider using this powerful technique for your harder goals. Then watch what happens. Share your results with another person.

13. Willpower is like a muscle that gets weaker the longer you use it at any given time. But if you exercise your willpower muscle for short periods of time day after day, it will eventually get stronger. That's why I encourage

everyone to work on their hardest and most important goals first thing in the morning when your willpower is the strongest, during what I call the **golden hours**. Did you try using the golden hours to focus on your priority goals? If so, what happened? If not, would you be willing to try using this technique. If not, why not?

14. Have you felt guilty about your procrastination in the past? Did reading this book help you realize your procrastination wasn't your fault? Now that you know the reasons you've put things off in the past, do you feel less guilty? If you still feel guilty, what would it take for you to let that go? What if you stopped procrastinating right this minute then started making up for lost time? Would you feel less guilty if your productivity skyrocketed because of the knowledge and skills you got from this book? Explain why or why not.

15. The flow state is a powerful way to get much more done in much less time. Describe a time when you went into flow. What were you doing? What was that like? Identify and share ways you could go into flow more often. What goal(s) could you focus on to help you enter a flow state?

16. Once you learn how to break bad habits and build healthy habits, your life will never be the same. Identify one bad habit you have broken in the past. What helped you change your habit? Name one healthy habit you still want to build. What techniques from the Chapter Seven on habits do you think would be the most likely to help you build that new habit? What is it about you that might make it hard to build your new habit? What could you do to help ensure your success? Share your answers to these questions.

17. What activities do you do that give you a dopamine rush and make you feel energized, exited, and happy? Which ones of those are healthy activities that add value to your life (like completing projects and learning new skills)? What unhealthy, high-dopamine substances would you like to stop using (for example, alcohol, sugar, caffeine, or marijuana)? What high-dopamine online behaviors would you like to cut back on or eliminate altogether (like social media and video games)? Review the techniques in Chapter Eight and decide on one strategy to try to help you change your behavior. Let your results from trying that strategy speak for themselves.

18. Changing your thoughts and behaviors can be challenging. To help you stay motivated, it's important to celebrate both your successes and your progress along the way to success. What are the ways you typically celebrate when you've earned a reward for your efforts? Buying yourself

a small gift? Enjoying a meal at your favorite restaurant? Getting a massage? List five ways you can celebrate that aren't too expensive or time consuming.

19. From reading this book, what is the most effective strategy you learned for how to stop procrastinating? What BIG, over-the-top goals do you think might finally be possible to achieve now that you have learned that strategy? What might hold you back from reaching those goals?

20. Having a Plan for Success and a Plan for Failure can make all the difference between success and failure with your goals. Do you tend to give up when your goals get hard? Or when you don't complete your goals as quickly as you think you should? How have you managed to keep going in the past? What additional techniques could you include in either your Plan for Success or your Plan for Failure that you would consider trying the next time you want to give up? If you get discouraged with one or more of your goals, remember the story of Diana Nyad and how it took her five attempts to make her famous swim from Cuba to Florida. She never gave up. She finally found a way. You can learn to be that determined with your own goals. Just keep going.

Permissions

I gratefully acknowledge the following authors who generously granted permission to use their copyrighted and previously published material. See the Notes section for additional information.

1. Piers Steel – *The Procrastination Equation*

2. Linda Sapadin – *How to Beat Procrastination in the Digital Age*

3. Christian Mickelsen – *Abundance Unleashed*

4. Nils Salzgeber – *Stop Procrastinating*

5. Kelly McGonigal – *The Willpower Instinct*

6. Deborah Sandella – *Goodbye, Hurt and Pain*

7. Brian Tracy – *Eat that Frog*

Notes

Within these Notes I have tried to reference my text and give ample credit to those whose work I have included. Despite my best efforts, however, I may have unintentionally omitted material that needs to be cited. There may also be information that is incorrect or that has changed over time. If you notice any omissions or incorrect citations, please contact me so I can correct them. You may email me at linda@lindagannaway. com. Thank you.

Chapter 1: Looking for Answers

Page

3   **with all kinds of limiting beliefs.** Mickelsen, Christian (2017). *Abundance unleashed*: *Open yourself to more money, love, health, and happiness n*ow. Hay House.

4   **those who are situational procrastinators** Ferrari, Joseph R. (2010). *Still procrastinating? The no-regrets guide to getting it done.* John Wiley & Sons. (page 166)

Chapter 2: The Good News About Procrastination

8   **severe memory problems—even Alzheimer's.** Bredesen, Dale E. (2017). *The end of Alzheimer's: The first program to prevent and reverse cognitive decline.* Penguin Random House. Bredesen reports good results with his program. Daniel Amen, author of numerous books including *Change Your Brain Every Day*, also reports positive results with dementia patients through his clinics and protocols.

11   **with our subconscious, internal conflicts.** This 80 percent is often quoted by experts in the field, including Mickelsen in *Abundance Unleashed* (Ibid), and Bruce Lipton (2016), *The biology of belief: Unleashing the power of consciousness, matter and miracles (10ᵗʰ anniversary edition).*

13   **than the students who were told nothing.** Wohl, Michael J.A., Pychyl, Timothy A., Bennett, Shannon H., (2010). I forgive myself, now I can study: How self-forgiveness for procrastinating can reduce future procrastination. *Personality and Individual Differences* 48, (pages 803-808).

14   **happier, healthier, and wealthier.** Steel, Piers (2011). *The procrastination equation: How to stop putting things off and start getting*

stuff done. HarperCollinsPublishers. (pages 84-85)

16   **you'll do what it takes.** Assaraf, John (2018). *Innercise: The new science to unlock yourbrain's hidden power.* Waterside Press. (pages 5-6). Note that Assaraf learned this adage from his mentor, Alan Brown.

16   **energized, excited, and happy.** Breuning, Loretta Graziano (2016). *Habits of a happy brain: Retrain your brain to boost your serotonin, dopamine, oxytocin, & endorphin levels.* Adams Media, an Imprint of Simon & Schuster. (pages 34-39)

25   **people who buy a book** Robbins, Anthony (1991). *Awaken the giant within: How to take immediate control of your mental, emotional, physical & financial destiny!* Fireside, a trademark of Simon & Schuster. (page 23)

Chapter 3: Why Do We Procrastinate?

29   *opportunity lost, and more. Much more."* Steel, *The procrastination equation.* Ibid (page 1)

29   **among the top reported goals— in the *world.*** Steel, *The procrastination equation.* Ibid (page 11)

29   **are more successful in overcoming it.** Ferrari, *Still procrastinating?* Ibid (page 7)

30   **outside of our conscious awareness.** Lipton, Bruce H. (2015). *The biology of belief: Unleashing the power of consciousness, matter & miracles.* Mountain of Love Productions. (page 229)

32   **to avoid uncomfortable emotions.** Lieberman, Charlotte (2019, March 25). Why you procrastinate (It has nothing to do with self-control). *New York Times* Smarter Living. https://www.nytimes.com/2019/03/25/smarter-living/why-you-procrastinate-it-has-nothing-to-do-with-self-control.html

37   **programmed into the subconscious."** Lipton, *The biology of belief.* Ibid (page 179)

40   **small and constricted.** See YouTube video. One week training with Wim Hof: Short documentary. https://www.youtube.com/watch?v=N-qvQGHHyOg. For more information on Wim Hof methods see WimHofmethod.com More documentation of moving out of our comfort zones can be found at https://www.herplanetearth.com/her-planet-earth-

news/ice-ice-baby-climbing-half-naked-with-wim-hof

42   **description of those styles.** Sapadin, Linda (2012). *How to beat procrastination in the digital age: 6 change programs for 6 personality styles*. PsychWisdom Publishing. (pages 22-24)

Chapter 4: Outsmart Impulsiveness

55   **I listen to him differently."** Namath, Joe with Mortimer, Sean and Yaeger, Don (2019). *All the way: My life in four quarters*. Little, Brown and Company, Hatchett Book Group. (page 171)

56   **all areas of their lives.** Dweck, Carol S. (2016). *Mindset: The new psychology of success*. Ballantine Books. (pages 5-7)

57   **which mindset we want to believe.** Dweck, *Mindset*. Ibid (page 16)

58   **because of impulsiveness.** Steel, *The Procrastination Equation*. Ibid (page 25)

60   **when dopamine is released.** Lehrer, Jonah (2010). *How we decide*. Mariner Books by Houghton Mifflin Harcourt. (page 34) Lehrer describes research that found the nucleus accumbens is the source of dopamine in the brain. This research is documented in Olds, James, and Milner, Peter (1954). Positive reinforcement produced by electrical stimulation of septal area and other regions of rat brain. *Journal of Comparative and Physiological Psychological Psychology* 47 (pages 419-427)

67   **use it at any given time.** McGonigal, Kelly (2012). *The willpower instinct: How self-control works, why it matters, and what you can do to get more of it*. Penguin Group. (page 79)

69   **rest of the day!** Tracy, Brian (2017). *Eat that frog: 21 great ways to stop procrastinating and get more done in less time*. Berrett-Koehler Publishers. (page 87)

70   **a classic in the field.** Lakein, Alan (1973). *How to get control of your time and your life*. Signet Book by Penguin Group.

74   **lift up your foot.** Sincero, Jen (2013). *You are a badass: How to stop doubting your greatness and start living an awesome life***.** Running Press, part of Hatchett Book Group. (page 149)

75   **success is inevitable.** Mickelsen, *Abundance Unleashed*. Ibid (page 116) This quote is similar to one that Mickelsen says often, "Your success is inevitable."

Chapter 5: Strategies to Stop Procrastinating

88   **to work through inner blocks.** Grace, Debbie Lynn. Grace made this suggestion during an online training after working with thousands of clients to help them release their inner blocks.

90   **seemed to be permanent.** Hawkins, David R. (2018). *Letting go: The pathway of surrender.* Hay House. (page xv)

93   **coaches around the world.** For more information on Mickelsen see www.coacheswithclients.com.

95   **over what could be years.** Hawkins, *Letting go.* Ibid (pages 9-10)

96   *Abundance Unleashed.* Mickelsen, *Abundance unleashed.* Ibid. You can also find more information about Mickelsen and his coaching practices at www.coacheswithclients.com.

99   **could change your life.** Curdy, Amy (2012). *Your body language may shape who you are.* ted.com/speakers/amy_curdy. TEDGlobal 2012.

103   **Olympics in Tokyo.** Brodsky, Samantha (2021, August 13). How Valarie Allman used affirmations before throwing Olympic discus gold. *Popsugar.* https://www.popsugar.com/fitness/valarie-allman-tokyo-olympics-discus-affirmations-interview-48460881

110   *Why? Why? Why?* Salzgeber, Nils (2017). *Stop procrastinating: A simple guide to hacking laziness, building self-discipline, and overcoming procrastination.* Nils Salzgeber at njlifehacks.com. (page 9)

110   **go crazy doing it!"** Salzgeber, *Stop Procrastinating.* Ibid (page 9)

110   *in full control of my life.* Salzgeber, *Stop Procrastinating.* Ibid (page 10)

110   *this way right now.* Salzgeber, *Stop Procrastinating.* Ibid (page 86)

115   **life turned around."** Nelson, Willie with Pipkin, Turk (2006). *The tao of willie: A guide to the happiness in your heart.* Gotham Books by Penguin Group. (page XII)

Chapter 6: Goal Setting that Accelerates Your Success

124   **January 19th to be exact.** Haden, Jeff (2020, January 3). A study of 800 million activities predicts most New Year's resolutions will be abandoned on January 19: How to create new habits that actually stick. Inc.com. https://www.inc.com/jeff-haden/a-study-of-800-million-activities-predicts-most-new-years-resolutions-will-be-abandoned-on-january-19-

how-you-cancreate-new-habits-that-actually-stick.html

124   **likely to be successful.** This figure comes from online training by Marisa Murgatroyd, an online coach and trainer to over 10,000 students. For more information see liveyourmessage.com

127   **by writing them down.** Keller, Gary with Papasan, Jay (2013). *The one thing: The surprisingly simple truth behind extraordinary results.* John Murry Learning. (page 154) This percentage is based on research by Gail Matthews at Dominican University of California. See Matthews, Gail, "The impact of commitment, accountability, and written goals on goal achievement" (2007). Psychology Faculty Presentations. 3.

129   **why they will give in."** McGonigal, *The willpower instinct.* Ibid (page 4)

133   **break the chain.** Newport, Cal (2016). *Deep work.* Grand Central Publishing, part of the Hachett Book Group. (pages 110-111)

133   **likely to achieve them.** Keller and Papasan, *The one thing.* Ibid (page 187). As before, Keller and Papasan reported this percentage from the research done by Gail Matthews at Dominican University of California.

134   **they would give to others.** Beatson, Brad, Lebofsky, Samantha, Roncinske, Kate, and Wojtala, Celine (2022, display until July 1, 2022). *Half their size: 20 years of real-life stories, inspiration & tips.* Special *People* Edition, 20th Anniversary Ed. Meredith Operations Corporation.

136   **even more motivation."** Beatson, Lebofsky, Roncinske, and Woitala (2022). *Half their size.* Ibid (page 13)

137   **triple whammy.** Mickelsen, Christian. Mickelsen discussed this during an online training after working with thousands of clients to help them release their inner blocks.

Chapter 7: The Advantages of Healthy Habits

148   **became "the one."** Elrod, Hal (2017). *The miracle morning: the not-so-obvious secret guaranteed to transform your life before 8 am.* Hal Elrod International.

149   **profoundly powerful formula.** Duhigg, Charles (2014). *The power of habit: Why we do what we do in life and business.* Random House.

151   *talk for ten minutes.* Duhigg, *The power of habit.* Ibid (page 297)

153   **avoiding unhappy chemicals."** Breuning, *Habits of a happy brain.* Ibid (page 22)

156   **they were "too tired."** Steel, *The procrastination equation.* Ibid (page 267)

158   **how long it took.** Rubin, Gretchen (2015). *Better than before: What I learned about making and breaking habits—to sleep more, quit sugar, procrastinate less, and generally build a happier life.* Broadway Books. (page 79) Rubin describes research done by Lally, Phillipa et al. (2010). How are habits formed: Modeling habit formation in the real world. *European Journal of Social Psychology* 40 (pages 998-1009)

159   **learn something instantly.** Breuning, *Habits of a happy brain.* Ibid (page 121)

164   ***will always feel deprived.*** Carr, Allen (2011). *Allen carr's easy way to stop smoking,* US ed. Allen Carr's Easyway (International). (page 3)

168   **easily lost the weight."** Beatson, Lebofsky, Roncinske, and Woitala, *Half their size.* Ibid (page 46)

168   **to alcoholism is resentment.** Anonymous (1976). *Alcoholics Anonymous: The story of how many thousands of men and women have recovered from alcoholism,* 3ʳᵈ ed. Alcoholics Anonymous World Service, Inc. (page 64) This book is often referred to as the *Big Book.*

169   **negative emotions.** Siegel, Bernie S. (1998). *Love, medicine and miracles: Lessons learned about self-healing from a surgeon's experience with exceptional patients.* HarperPerennial.

169   **molecules . . . (in the body)."** Breuning, *Habits of a happy brain.* Ibid (page 121)

169   **anchors in body memory."** Sandella, Deborah (2016). *Goodbye, hurt &pain. 7 simple steps for health, love, and success.* Conari Press, an imprint of RedWheel/Weiser. (page 79) Sandella's work draws from that of Rick Hanson with Richard Mendius (2009) in their book, *Buddha's Brain: The Practical Neuroscience of Happiness, Love & Wisdom.* Sandella's work is further supported by that of Bessel A. Van der Kolk (2015) in his book, *The Body Keeps the Score: Brain, Mind, and Body in the Healing of Trauma.*

169   **out-of-control and anxious."** Sandella, *Goodbye, hurt & pain.* Ibid (page 80)

172   **control over them."** Van der Kolk, Bessel A. (2015). *The body keeps the score: Brain, mind, and body in the healing of trauma.* Penguin

Books. (page 210)

172   **in my chest.'"** Van der Kolk, *The body keeps the score*. Ibid (pages 210-211)

173   **back of this book.** The Tapping Foundation Solution video of interviews with some of those traumatized by the Sandy Hook shooting. On Facebook see https://www.facebook.com/watch/?v=827816270741749

173   **lead to faster results.** This blog post by Nick Ortner contains updates on the Sandy Hook Project conducted by The Tapping Foundation Solution. See https://www.thetappingsolution.com/blog/tapping-solution-foundation-update-newtown/

173   **by author Dawson Church,** Church, Dawson (2018). *Mind to matter: The astounding science of how your brain creates material reality*. Hay House. This research study and many others on Tapping (EFT) can be found at https://eftuniverse.com/research-studies/

Chapter 8: Protect Your Priorities from Too Much Screen Time

180   **irritability and depression.** Lembke, Anna (2021). *Dopamine nation: Finding balance in the age of indulgence.* Penguin Random House. (pages 56-57)

180   **cocaine show similar impairments.** Lembke, *Dopamine nation.* Ibid (page 50) This similarity is also reported by an internet addiction (IAD) recovery program, Talbott Recovery (talbottcampus.com, How internet addiction affects . . .) in their statement: "IAD alters the volume of the brain. The brain changes are similar to those produced by alcohol and cocaine addiction. IAD shrinks the brain's gray and white matter fibers which results in changes to emotional processing and brain functioning."

181   **spend on their phones.** Plumhoff, Katherine (2022, display until July 2022). The attack of the phones: Spending too much time on your devices? Here's how to realistically break your social media habit. Special *Health* Edition on Understanding Addiction, Meredith Corporation. (page 31)

183   **specialist Kimberly Young.** The late Kimberly Young founded the Center for Internet Addiction in 1995 to provide education and treatment for internet addiction. See netaddiction.com for more information. Her self-scoring Internet Addiction Test consists of 20 questions and can be found at www.iitk.ac.in/counsel/resources/IATManual.pdf

183   **a simple yes or no.** These questions can indicate internet addiction and

are similar to questions listed on netaddiction.com (see reference above)

185   **the self-regulation you have."** Alter, Adam (2017). *Irresistible: The rise of addictive technology and the business of keeping us hooked.* Penguin Books. (page 3)

185   **with Steve Jobs and Bill Gates** Price, *How to break up with your phone.* Ibid (pages 21-22)

190   **the more lonely they feel.** Twinge, Jean M. (2017). *iGen: Why today's super-connected kids are growing up less rebellious, more tolerant, less happy—and completely unprepared for adulthood.* Ataria, an imprint of Simon and Schuster. (page 80)

190   **self-criticism, and low self-esteem.** Price, Catherine (2018). *How to break up with your phone.* Ten Speed Press. (page 34)

191   **read something like this:** Newport, Cal (2019). *Digital minimalism: Choosing a focused life in a noisy world.* Penguin Business. (page 69)

194   ***How to Break Up with Your Phone.*** Price, *How to break up with your phone.* Ibid

195   **Ask yourself these questions.** Lembke, Anna (2021). *Dopamine Nation: Finding balance in the age of indulgence.* Penguin Random House. (page 77)

195   **months at a time.** Alter, *Irresistible,* Ibid (pages 251-254)

196   **function at its best.** Julson, Erica (2023, July 10). 10 Best ways to increase dopamine levels naturally. *Healthline.* https://www.healthline.com/nutrition/how-to-increase-dopamine

198   **(You Will Too)."** Becker, Alex. This made me quit alcohol forever (You will too). This YouTube video by Alex Becker can be found at https://www.youtube.com/watch?v=tEWweaj_Zyo

199   **will often go away.** Carr, Allen (2014). *The easy way to control alcohol.* Arcturus Publishing Limited. (page 170)

Chapter 9: It's About Time

203   **owned a smartphone.** Twinge, *iGen.* Ibid (page 4)

204   **that of a goldfish!** Alter, *Irresistible.* Ibid (page 28 Alter describes research conducted in 2000 by Microsoft Canada, Consumer Insights, Attention Spans, Spring 2015, advertising.microsoft.com/en/WWDocs/

User/display/cl/researchreport/31966/en/microsoft-attention-spans-research-report.pdf.

205 **throughout the whole day.** The time lost when you shift your attention away from a task is also referred to as task switching and includes multitasking. The research showing that it takes 25 minutes to get back to full concentration has been widely shared by researcher Gloria Mark. For example, see The science of our attention spans with professor Gloria Mark. Cambride ThinkLab. https://www.youtube.com/watch?v=ebj_-QmCTbk More information can be found in Mark, Gloria (2023). *Attention span: Finding focus for a fulfilling life.* William Collins, HarperCollins Publishers.

205 **complete these valuable goals.** Tracy, *Eat that frog.* Ibid (page 94)

205 **now reached 57 percent.** Kerai, Alex (July 21, 2023). Cell phone usage statistics: Mornings are for notifications. *Reviews.org.* https://www.reviews.org/mobile/cell-phone-addiction/

206 **focus when we need to.** Price, *How to break up with your phone.* Ibid (pages 52-53)

208 **Calm is a superpower.** This quote is often attributed to Bruce Lee.

210 **further illustrates my point.** This well-known Taoist farmer story has several versions. I have written it here from memory, but the story is the same. You can find a longer version and the meaning of the story at https://mindfulness.com/mindful-living/are-these-bad-times-or-good-times-the-story-of-the-zen-farmer

216 **what you don't want."** This quote is attributed to several authors but most often to Robert Downey Jr.

217 **self-conscious, and depressed.** Price, *How to break up with your phone.* Ibid (page 11)

219 **which became a bestseller.** Csikszentmihalyi, Mihaly (1990). *Flow: The psychology of optimal experience.* HarperPerennial.

221 **anandamide, and serotonin.** Kotler, Steven (2014). *The rise of superman: Decoding the science of ultimate human performance.* Amazon Publishing. (pages 66-68)

222 **three steps described below.** Kotler, *The rise of superman.* Ibid. (pages 114-117)

224 **by 490 percent. Wow.** See www.flowresearchdirective.com, a website for flow research and training.

225   **here's how it works.** Robbins, *Awaken the giant within.* Ibid (page 165) This technique is similar to those described by Robbins on how to change submodalities (auditory, visual and kinesthetic) in order to change emotional intensity. This process is based on neurolinguistic programming (NLP) and was first introduced by John Grinder and Richard Bandler in their books *The Structure of Magic,* Vols 1 and 2.

226   **international best seller.** Tracy, *Eat that frog.* Ibid (page 29)

228   **about five hours a day.** Graziosi, Dean (2019). *Millionaire success habits: The gateway to wealth & prosperity.* Dean Graziosi. (page 232)

229   **your ultimate priority.** Canfield, Jack with Switzer, Janet (2015). *The success principles: How to get from where you are to where you want to be*, 10ᵗʰ anniversary ed. HarperCollins. (pages 217-218)

230   **S.A.V.E.R.S.,** Elrod, *The miracle morning.* Ibid (page 92)

231   **start to reflect that growth.** Elrod, *The miracle morning.* Ibid (page 53)

231   **meditation and reading.** Badziag, Rafael (2019). *The billion dollar secret: 20 principles of billionaire wealth and success.* Panoma Press. (pages 102-110)

237   **differences down the road.** Hardy, Darren (2010). *The compound effect: Jumpstart your income, your life, your success.* Da Capo Press, Perseus Books Group.

244   *than not to complete them.* Tracy, *Eat that frog.* Ibid (page 4)

246   **urge to smoke.** Price, *How to break up with your phone.* Ibid (pages 70-71) Price describes mindfulness research by Brewer, A. et al (2011). Mindfulness training for smoking cessation: Results from a randomized controlled trial. *Drug and Alcohol Dependence* 119, nos 1-2. (pages 72-80)

248   **alone with their thoughts.** Jarvis, Paul (2018). *Company of one: Why staying small is the next big thing for business.* Mariner Books, Houghton Mifflin Harcourt. (page xii) Jarvis describes a study by Wilson, Timothy D., Reinhard, David A., Westgate, Erin C., Gilbert, Daniel T., and Shaked, Adi (July 4, 2014). Just think: The challenges of the disengaged mind. Science 345, no 6192 (pages 75-77)

248   **ongoing, natural high.** Pert, Candace B. (1997). *Molecules of emotion: Why you feel the way you feel.* Schribner. (page 130)

249   **illness and disease.** Lipton, *The biology of belief.* Ibid (page 155)

Chapter 10: You Were Born to Shine

256   ***that most frightens us.*** Williamson, Marianne (1992). *A return to love: Reflections on the principles of a course in miracles.* HarperCollins Publishers. (page 165)

258   ***automatically liberates others.*** Williamson, *A return to love.* Ibid (page 165)

262   **rang true for me.** O'Connell, Lauren. Aging backwards/aging well – How and why I quit coffee – 40 years old. Youtube, https://www.youtube.com/watch?v=qPq04lBtCEc&t=507s

263   **"The one you feed."** This well-known story of the two wolves has several different versions. I have told the story here, mostly in my own words, but referencing a version that is included in Keller and Papasan's book, *The one thing.* Ibid (page 211)

267   **and an outer purpose.** Tolle, Eckhard (2005). *A new earth: Awakening to your life's purpose.* Plume, part of the Penguin Group. (page 269)

275   **they regret the most.** Ware, Bronnie (2012). *The top five regrets of the dying: A life transformed by the dearly departing.* Hay House.

Index

Acknowledgements

The information in this book came from a wide variety of sources, and I'm grateful for each one. These sources included my mentors and coaches, as well as authors, researchers in psychology and brain science, family members, friends, colleagues, complete strangers, and my university students and coaching clients. They also included my intuitive epiphanies and life experiences, especially the many years I procrastinated, and the successes and failures I had along the way. Each source contributed to the lessons I needed to learn to put this book together and offer it to you.

First of all, to the Fresno State University students who were in my classes and individual and group counseling sessions. Thank you so much for what you taught me. Your candor and courage in sharing your struggles and successes made you excellent teachers, and you inspired me every day.

To Dennis Nef for giving me the opportunity to work with thousands of students in the freshman orientation classes that were offered at Fresno State. Those classes helped me get a meta-level perspective on our students' learning processes and to clearly see the differences between situational and chronic procrastinators.

To the people who have attended my talks and workshops and so freely discussed their experiences with procrastination. I may have been doing a lot of the talking, but I was learning so much from you.

To my family—my late parents, Sarah and Jim Gannaway, and to my sisters, Sharon Gannaway and Vivian Gannaway Walker (I call her VS). How was I so fortunate to be born into a family with you? I can't express how much I appreciate your love and support, your values and guidance, and for all you helped me learn. Again, my apologies for all the times I made you wait on me!

To my sister, VS, for using your excellent editing skills with this entire book, for your astute understanding of the concepts, for your honest feedback, your rock-solid, ongoing support of my writing process in general, which has meant more than you could know, and for listening to my countless experiences while I was writing. Your intention and the energy, knowledge, and skills you contributed to this book were immensely helpful. I also appreciated your keen eye and valuable insights and suggestions on the book cover design.

To the late CJ Collins for your critiques, professional expertise, and limitless generosity and patience in editing the first several chapters of this book, through *nine* revisions. Your input was essential in those early drafts when I was trying to establish the tone and explain the concepts of what was to follow. After your passing, I felt your spirit with me every step of the way as I continued to write.

To the late Janice Stevens for your unwavering support of me and my writing and for teaching writing classes in ways that allowed each class member to shine. I attended your Writing for Publication class for four years when I was writing my first book. You and the other students listened to me read every word and gave me your honest and caring feedback. Although I didn't attend the class when I was writing this book, as I wrote it, I could literally hear, inside my head, the comments you would probably make. What a welcome and appreciated surprise to realize I had internalized your voices. All of the critiques and suggestions you offered on my first book definitely helped make this book better.

Many thanks to these members of the Writing for Publication class: Richard Bailey, the late Jim Benelli, Robert Eiland, David Elkin, Mary Eurgubian, Don Farris, Veronica Giolli, Lucia Hammar, Earlene Holguin, Beverly Horsley, Gus Knittel, Sue Bonner Martin, Terry Meechan, Jim Mobley, Tom Morton, Linda Robertson, Pat Shanley, the late Chuck Soley, Fran Thomas, and the late Franz Weinschenk. A special thanks to Hank Palmer for believing in me and my message and for regularly cheering me on. And to the late CJ Collins, my heartfelt thanks for your friendship, your support as a fellow writer, and for consistently questioning the content of my book. Your honesty on both books was such a gift.

To my friends and colleagues, especially: Gena Gechter, for team-teaching a procrastination class with me and for giving me the concept of a successful procrastinator; Sue Tarr for your support as a fellow author and for your spiritual inspiration; Arlene Bireline for your core values and for your many years of friendship and professional mentorship; Kathy Winter for your friendship and love and for always being there; Minnie Loftus for your love and support, which started when we were in high school; Elizabeth Mason, for your understanding and enthusiastic encouragement for my writing; Janeil Swarthout for your feedback on my first book, which helped me decide to write this one; Erich Gross for your comments about flow and for all your help with my side projects; and to Gary Funk and Fabienne Buckle, for being such supportive next-door neighbors.

An important thanks goes to the Muse, my intuition, the source of all creativity, and my connection to the Inner Witness. Thank you for your guidance, your wisdom, and for pulling me out of one pinch after another when I felt overwhelmed while writing this book and when my thoughts ran into a dead end. All I needed to do was be quiet and listen inside for your voice.

Thanks to 100 Covers for the cover design.

And a special thanks to Michael at MGF for the interior formatting and cartoon character customizations.

To the coaches, mentors and authors who guided me through the content of this book. What you have helped me learn has been invaluable. My deep gratitude to all of you, including Christian Mickelsen, Linda Sapadin, Piers Steel, Deborah Sandella, Loretta Graziano Breuning, Brian Tracy, Jack Canfield, Dean Graziosi, John Assaraf, Tony Robbins, Jane Burka, Lenora Yuen, David Hawkins, Nils Salzgeber, Daniel Amen, Charles Duhigg, James Clear, Bruce Lipton, Carol Dweck, Kelly McGonigal, Marisa Murgatroyd, Debbie Lynn Grace, B.J. Fogg, and Alex Becker. I hope this book helps all of you help more people through what you have shared with me.

A final thanks goes to you, the reader. Thank you for sticking with this book until the end, for the belief you've had in your own ability to change, for understanding that overcoming procrastination is a goal worth pursuing, and for the actions you take to improve your life. You inspire me! I applaud and congratulate you for your efforts and wish you unlimited abundance, happiness, and success.

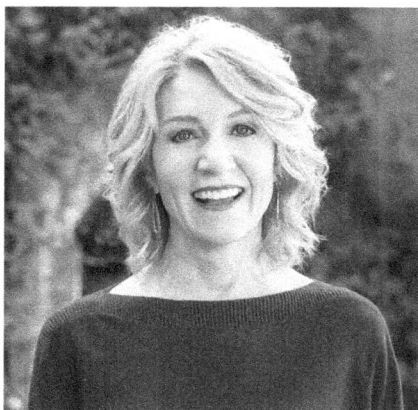

About the Author

After procrastinating for much of her life, Dr. Linda Gannaway finally broke free from the beliefs and habits that had kept her stuck. She's now on a mission to help others learn how to do the same. Her experiences and education have provided the foundation to share science-based strategies that help people get more done in less time.

Linda received her doctorate, an Ed.D. in counseling, from the University of Arkansas, Fayetteville. She also completed a predoctoral internship in counseling and clinical psychology at the University of Texas at Austin. She worked more than twenty-five years at several universities as a personal counselor, an administrator, and an instructor, teaching classes to thousands of students on procrastination, time management, stress management, and goal setting. Her students helped her see patterns of unhealthy choices people can make—often based on long-held, negative beliefs about themselves—that can block them from achieving the success they want.

While writing her book on procrastination, Linda found that in this digital age, the main avoidance activity people use when they procrastinate is spending too much time on their phones. Realizing she was addicted to screen time, she learned to overcome her own internet addiction by practicing strategies in her book for developing healthy habits around being online.

Linda lives in California's Central Valley. She enjoys speaking, writing, training, and life coaching.

www.ingramcontent.com/pod-product-compliance
Lightning Source LLC
Chambersburg PA
CBHW031117020426
42333CB00012B/115